Yogacise™

Vimla Lalvani

THE NEW CONCEPT IN FITNESS

Yogacise ™

Vimla Lalvani

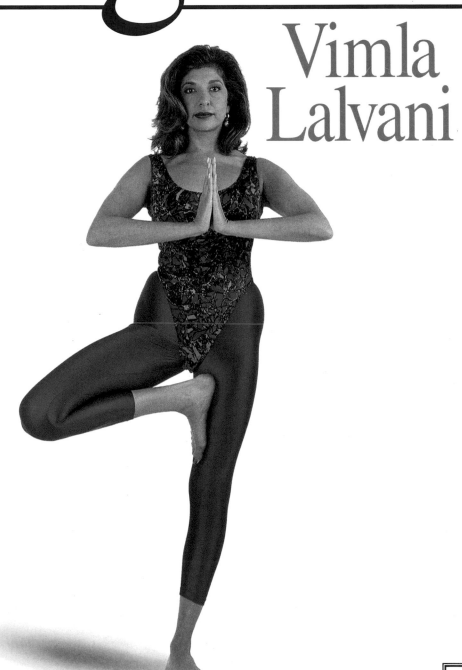

HAMLYN

This edition first published in Great Britain in 1995 by
Hamlyn, an imprint of Reed Consumer Books,
part of Reed International Books Limited,
Michelin House, 81 Fulham Road, London SW3 6RB
and Auckland, Melbourne, Singapore and Toronto

Licensed from Simitar Entertainment
Copyright © 1994 Revelation Film Ltd
Design © 1994 Reed International Books Ltd

Yogacise™ is a registered trademark.

ISBN 0 600 58244 2

A CIP catalogue record for this book
is available from the British Library.

Printed and bound by New Interlitho, Italy

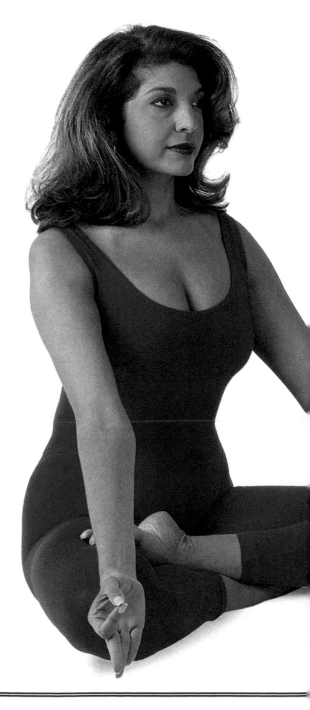

Contents

Foreword

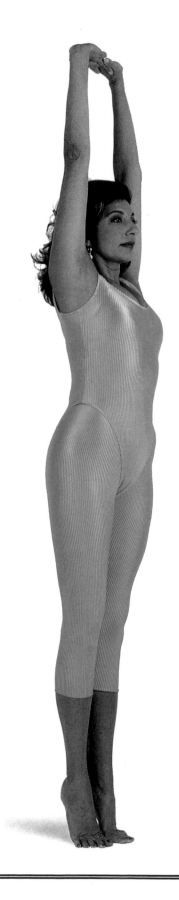

I have been teaching *Hatha* Yoga for more than 20 years in both Britain and the United States of America. During this time I have instructed over 1000 students of all ages, with different vocations and from all walks of life – artists, models, businessmen, housewives, secretaries, teenagers and pensioners. The popularity of Yoga is largely due to its wide range of therapeutic effects on both the mind and the body. When fully mastered, *Hatha* Yoga is a means by which the restless mind is calmed and physical and mental energy is directed into constructive channels.

Yoga is not a religion but a philosophy of life. It is also a discipline with a scientific background. It is universal and timeless and as relevant today as it was when it was first developed 2000 years ago. In fact, it is the perfect way to maintain a balanced outlook in the face of pressures from modern-day living.

Yogacise combines the ancient principles of *Hatha* Yoga with modern stretch techniques. Some people are put off Yoga by its mystical connotations and by the fact that they imagine it involves being tied up in knots, but hopefully they will find Yogacise far more accessible. It teaches you how to concentrate and focus your mind, improve your muscle tone and invigorate your internal organs. It also teaches you how to breathe correctly and how to attain perfect posture, enabling you to increase your energy levels. The results will be dramatic. You will develop a perfectly toned body, a positive outlook on life and a peaceful mind.

I hope this book will be a source of inspiration and set you on a path of self-discovery. So, go ahead, and discover the potential within your mind and body.

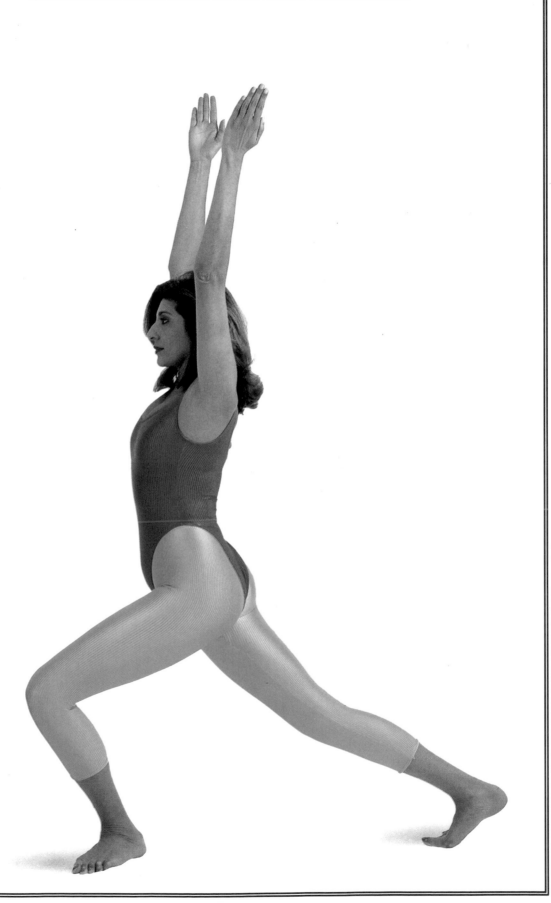

Introduction

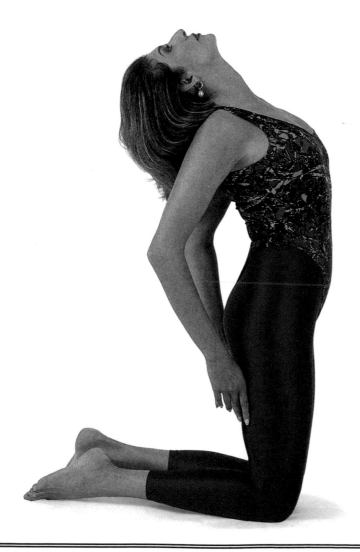

The benefits of Yogacise

Yogacise is the new concept in fitness that combines *Hatha* Yoga techniques with modern stretch exercises. Experts agree that stretching is the best way to achieve top-to-toe fitness and combined with Yoga, with its centuries-old system, Yogacise provides one of the safest, most effective ways to exercise.

This book demonstrates simple ways to improve breathing techniques and posture and contains over 50 body-conditioning exercises that will improve flexibility, stamina and muscle tone. Stretching is the most natural way to release tension in the muscle groups and when combined with correct breathing destresses the nervous system and increases energy levels. You will find that Yogacise produces powerful results: an invigorated body, increased stamina, improved muscle tone and a feeling of total harmony and well-being.

The contribution of traditional Yoga

Yoga is a Sanskrit word meaning 'the union of mind and body'. According to ancient texts it is a science that allows us to live a harmonious life through the control of the mind and body. *Hatha* Yoga is about combining energy from *Ha,* the masculine sun energy and *Tha*, the feminine moon energy. Together they balance the body and produce harmony and equilibrium so you do not suffer mood swings or depression. You feel on an even keel and ready to cope with life. The main principle of Yoga is that before you can train your mind to reach a higher consciousness you must first discipline your body. *Hatha* Yoga is the first stage because it concentrates on the physical. Deep stretches and fluid movements unblock energy, increase stamina and improve muscle tone. Combined with correct breathing, Yoga will increase vitality and energy levels as well as discipline the mind.

How to use this book

The book is divided into five 10–20-minute workouts that can be interchanged depending on the time of day and how busy you are. Rise and Shine and Energizer are good morning workouts while De-stress is perfect for the evening. Classical and Ultimate Stretch can be performed at any time. Always perform the exercises in the order in which they appear within each workout as each section has been carefully designed to warm and stretch muscles, ligaments and tendons in a particular order. It is a good idea to read through all the instructions for an exercise before you begin so that you can pace yourself accordingly.

Yogacise compared with other forms of exercise

The main differences between Yogacise and other forms of exercise are the emphasis on correct breathing and the length of time each position is held. Holding a position for 5 seconds or more allows a graceful flow of energy and gives the mind a chance to focus while improving the physical body. Just as water flows through an open tap, so energy flows into the relaxed muscles. As various joints are twisted, blood vessels are pulled and stretched and blood is equally distributed through the body. All Yogacise exercises are based on a formula of stretching, relaxation, deep breathing and increasing circulation and concentration. Yogacise encourages total body health and you will soon be well on the way to a new lifestyle.

Yogacise is non-competitive. Take it gently and listen to your body. Do not be discouraged if you cannot achieve the final position for some time – Yogacise is a discipline so continued practice will bring results. The main difference between an intermediate and an advanced student of Yoga is the length of time they are able to hold the positions. Challenge yourself by setting goals to help you progress.

Explanation of terms

The Sanskrit terms *asana*, *chakra*, *prana* and *pranayama* are used throughout the book to describe classical concepts: *Asanas* are the recognized Yoga postures. *Chakras* are the seven energy centers within the body. *Prana* is vital energy and the solar plexus is like a storage battery supplying *prana* energy to the whole body.

Energy moves in different patterns through the body. Circular energy flows around the body and generates a feeling of flying. Examples of this pattern are found in the Standing Bow, Head to Knee and Letter T, to name a few. There are also 'grounding' exercises that take the energy from the earth in a linear pattern to the top of your head, such as the Eagle and Knee Bends 1, 2 and 3. These keep your focus on practical issues and help to give you a realistic outlook on life.

Pranayama is the science of breathing correctly and relates to breathing techniques to increase lung capacity, balance energies and focus your concentration. At an advanced level these techniques form the basis of Yoga meditation.

The 'lotus' position and 'half-lotus' position are associated with *pranayama* and meditation. This pose is very important when students sit for long periods during breathing exercises and meditation. First of all, this erect position of the spine will still retain its natural curve. Secondly, training the body to sit motionless reduces the metabolic rate. When the body is still the mind becomes free from all physical and psychological disturbances. A straight spine also creates a steady flow of nerve current through the body.

'Centering' the body is to focus on balancing your physical and mental state. Concentrate on the solar plexus and you will feel the harmony and inner peace of total balance.

'Opening the chest' is another term used in this book. It involves lifting the chest and pushing your shoulders down to create a positive outlook. Combined with a steady and direct gaze, it will show the world you are ready to face life with strength and confidence.

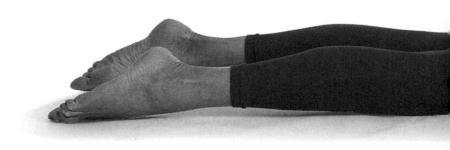

Important safety guidelines

* These exercises are designed for people in normal health. As with any fitness program, if you feel unfit, are recovering from any injury or illness, are pregnant, have high blood pressure or suffer from any other medical disorder, consult your doctor before embarking on these exercises.

* Always follow the recommended warm-up before attempting the main exercises. You can loosen up your muscles even more by taking a shower first.

* It is important to follow the given order of the exercises within each section and to read through each exercise before starting.

* Never rush the movements or force or jerk your body in any direction. Stop immediately if you feel any sharp pain or strain. Remember that the final pose in any exercise is usually the most challenging and with practice, you will become more flexible.

* Let your deep breathing relax your body and allow the stretched muscles and ligaments carry more energy to the muscle fibers.

* In many positions you will notice that the knee remains straight. Do not hyper-extend the knee but lift the muscle above the kneecap to avoid strain or injury.

* Do not attempt Yogacise on a full stomach – allow an interval of one hour after a light meal and four hours after a heavy meal.

* Wear loose, comfortable clothing.

* Exercise in a warm, well-ventilated place.

* Remain barefoot so you are able to grip with your toes. Make sure you practice on an even, non-slip surface. You may find it more comfortable to use a mat for the floor exercises.

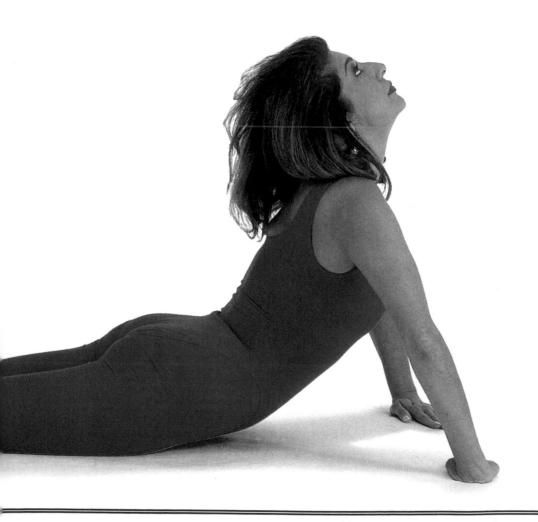

Lifestyle

Moderation is the key to a healthy, balanced lifestyle, and if the mind and body are in harmony, there is no inner need for excesses. This is not a question of abstinence but a matter of controlling your habits and urges. You do not have to become a vegetarian and give up smoking and drinking alcohol overnight. You will discover that if you practice Yogacise, you will gradually change of your own accord by eating, smoking and drinking less. Your body will reach its optimum weight and your temper will be even.

You will find your outlook on life is more positive. You will no longer experience serious mood swings or depression. As your concentration improves, you will be more organized and find yourself able to handle several tasks at the same time equally well.

Yoga philosophy offers people a scientific way of transcending their problems and suffering. It does not conflict with any religion or faith and can be practiced by anyone who is sincere and willing to discipline their life and search for truth. Little effort will bring immense returns like wisdom, strength and peace. As your awareness of your body increases, you will learn to listen to your 'higher self'. *Hatha* Yoga is the first step to spiritual enlightenment. However, the philosophy states that before you can discipline your mind and master the techniques of meditation, you must first discipline your body.

Many pupils of Yogacise find that they develop an interest in their own spiritual development, others do not. While some people concentrate only on balancing the mind and body, others find that they develop an insatiable need to go further. Each person is different and should follow their own inclinations.

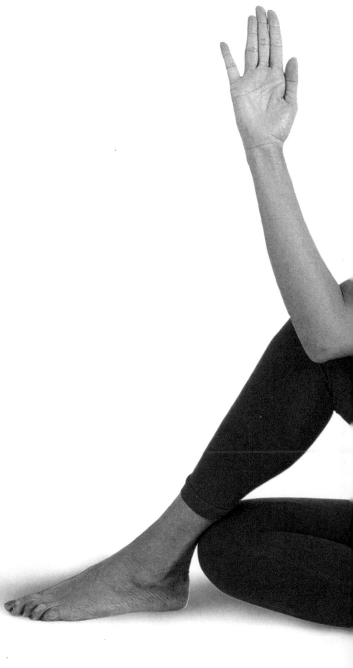

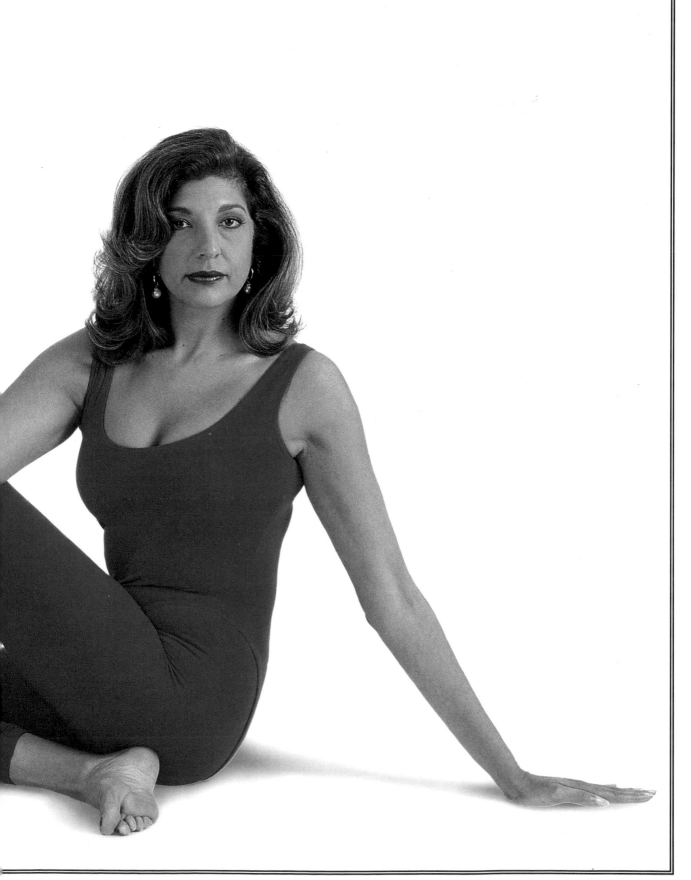

Posture

Most people do not realize how important it is to stand and sit correctly. Bad posture is the main cause of chronic back pain and contributes to painful ailments such as slipped discs and sciatica. Invariably, people with bad posture lack energy and vitality. Their chests are slumped, and they do not breathe correctly as they only use a small portion of their lungs.

Yogacise is designed to stretch the spine constantly and build the muscles in the lower back, enabling you to achieve perfect posture. You may think you are standing or sitting correctly, but you may not understand your own body alignment. Indeed, pregnancy or weight gain or loss can unbalance you.

Whether you are standing, kneeling or sitting, imagine that a string is pulling you upward from the top of your head. Push your shoulder blades down and lift the chest naturally. When you are in perfect posture, you will feel 'centered'. It is rather like placing building blocks on top of each other. If they are not evenly placed, they will tumble down.

The exercises in this book frequently refer to 1st and 2nd position. In 1st position stand with your feet together and touching each other. Open the toes evenly and press your heels down. In 2nd position stand with your feet approximately 30cm (1ft) apart. The feet should be positioned below the hips with toes pointing forward.

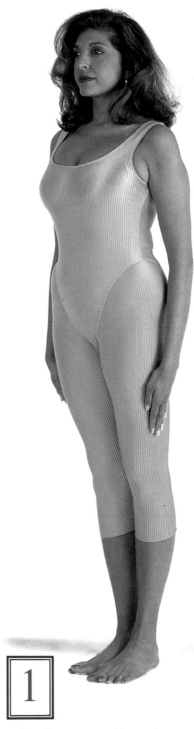

Stand as tall as you can with your feet together, keeping your shoulders down and your stomach and tail-bone tucked in.

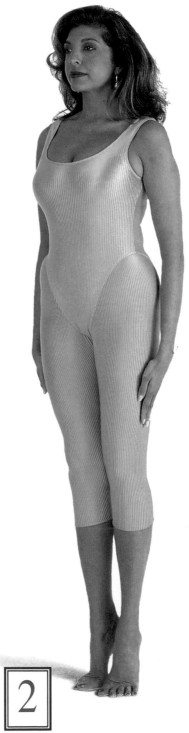

Raise your heels and balance on your toes. If you do not fall forward or backward you are in perfect posture.

POSTURE

In Steps 1 and 2 below, test yourself for perfect standing posture.
(In Step 1, it is important to distribute your weight evenly.) Steps 3
and 4 demonstrate correct posture when kneeling and sitting.

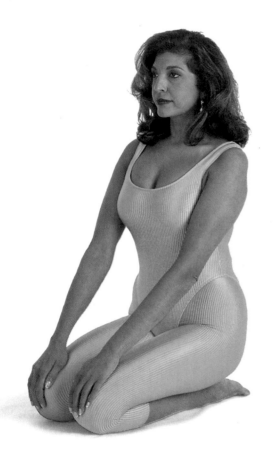

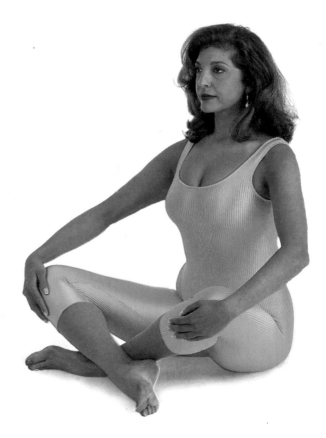

3

*Sit on your heels and place your hands
on your knees. Now raise your spine,
straightening your elbows.*

4

*Sitting cross-legged, lift the spine as far as
you can. This centers your balance, creating
a positive mental attitude.*

Breathing

Breathing correctly is an integral part of Yogacise. All the movements you perform, if they are to be beneficial, require correct breathing. To breathe correctly means breathing through the nose from the diaphragm, unless instructed otherwise (as in Nerve Soother on page 122 where you exhale through the mouth). As we exhale from the diaphragm, our lung capacity increases and more oxygen reaches the bloodstream. This rejuvenates and revitalizes the cells, resulting in increased energy levels and a strong, healthy body.

When you are breathing correctly, you should breathe fluidly and evenly like a wave in the sea, flowing in natural rhythm. Take a few seconds to inhale and exhale. As you inhale the stomach extends outward and as you exhale the stomach contracts inward. As you practice you will notice that your breathing pattern increases in depth and duration and becomes very quiet.

In Yogacise, you will use breathing techniques, known in Sanskrit as *pranayama*, that will balance the energies and focus the mind. Within the body there are seven energy centers known as *chakras*.

1

Place both hands on your stomach just below the waist and inhale slowly and evenly through your nose from the diaphragm. Feel your stomach distend as the diaphragm expands. Do not move your chest and shoulders.

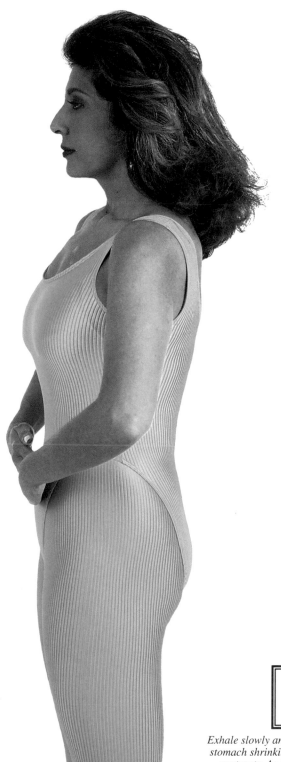

Pranayama techniques unlock blockages so the stream of energy flows smoothly from the base of the spine up to the top of the head to connect with the universal energy. When the subtle *prana,* or energy, is controlled, the body also comes under the mind's control and all imbalances are destroyed. If the body is strong and healthy, the energy flows freely.

Alternative Nostril Breathing (see page 105) shows you the difference between the masculine and feminine principle of energy. The right nostril is stronger, more fiery and more intense, ie. masculine; the left is softer, cooler and more gentle, i.e. feminine. This technique combines the masculine and feminine energies to balance the entire system.

Deep breathing techniques act like a tranquilizer, calming the nervous system. The deeper you breathe, the stronger the effect and the more able you are to combat stress. *Pranayama* not only teaches willpower and self-control but also improves concentration and encourages spiritual development.

2

Exhale slowly and evenly and feel your stomach shrinking as your diaphragm contracts. As in Step 1, remember to resist moving your chest and shoulders.

Warm-up

Many injuries are caused to the limbs, tendons and muscles when the body is not properly warmed-up and loosened. This Warm-up isolates different parts of the body and slowly stretches any stiffness out in preparation for most of the exercises that follow. If you are exercising first thing in the morning, however, it is better to use the Total Body Warm-up in the Rise and Shine section (see page 26).

While following the sequence, try to keep the muscles in your stomach and buttocks tight and distribute your weight evenly between your toes and heels. It is also a good idea to pay special attention to the instructions for inhaling and exhaling to allow a correct flow of energy through the body.

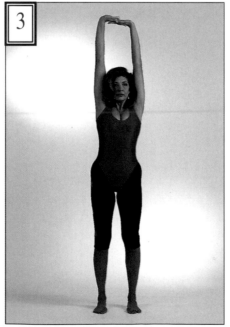

Breathing normally, stand tall with feet together in 1st position and arms slightly raised at your sides.

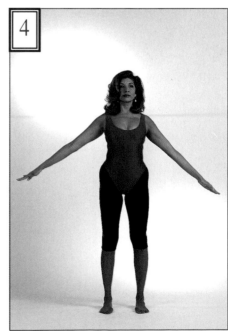

Place feet in 2nd position 15–20cm (6–8in) apart. Clasp your hands in front of you. Start to inhale as you raise your arms.

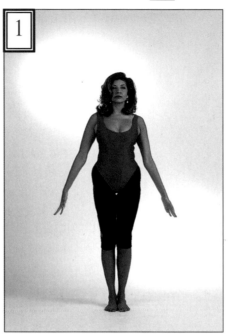

Still inhaling, stretch up, raising your arms as high as you can. Tighten your buttock muscles and tuck your tail-bone in.

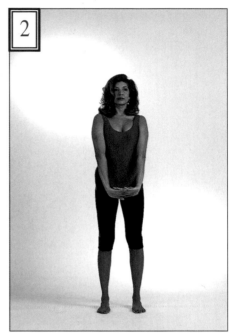

Exhale and release your arms to the sides. Lift your knees by using the muscle above the kneecaps.

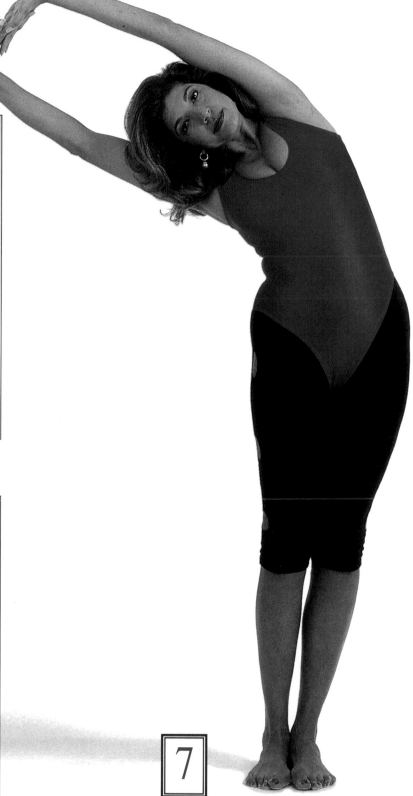

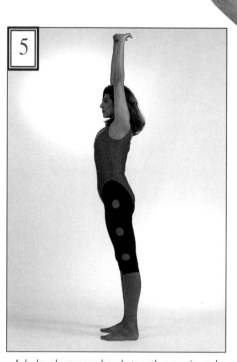

Inhale, clasp your hands together again and raise your arms as high as you can above your head, as in Step 3.

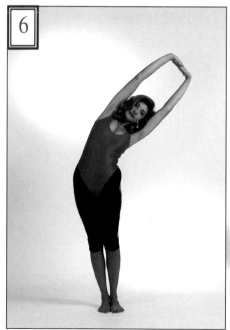

Bring feet together. Exhale and stretch to the left. Keep your hips square to increase the stretch. Hold for 10 seconds.

Inhale and stretch back up through 1st position. Exhale and stretch over to the right. Hold for 10 seconds, breathing normally.

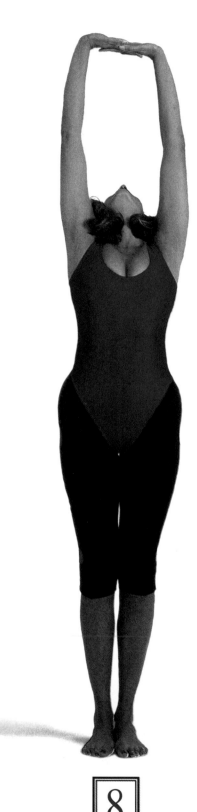

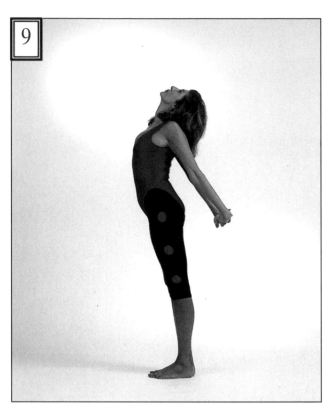

Exhale, take your arms down to your sides then behind your back and clasp your hands. Inhale. This releases tension from the back.

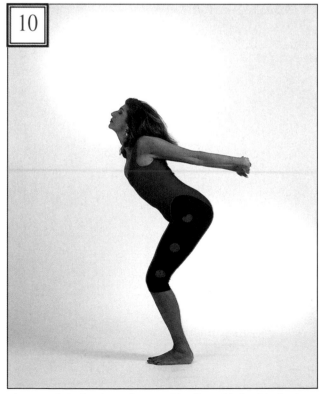

As you exhale, bend your knees and leading with the chin, begin to stretch forward slowly.

8

Inhale and stretch up again, keeping palms up. Look up to your hands, as you release tension in the neck and shoulders.

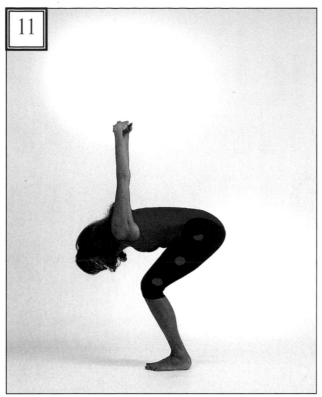

Stretching your arms straight up helps to eliminate the curve from your spine and enables you to achieve the flat back position.

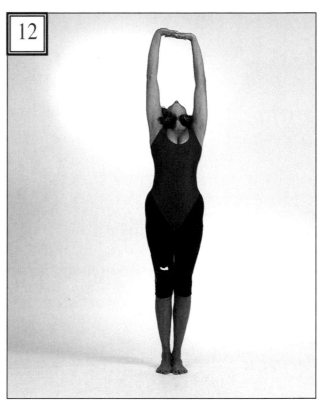

Breathing normally, straighten your legs, release your hands and stand upright. Inhale and stretch your arms as in Step 8.

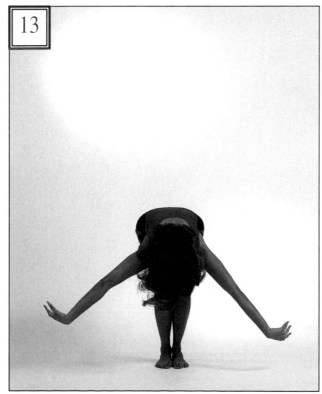

Exhale and bend your knees. Release your hands and relax your body forward.

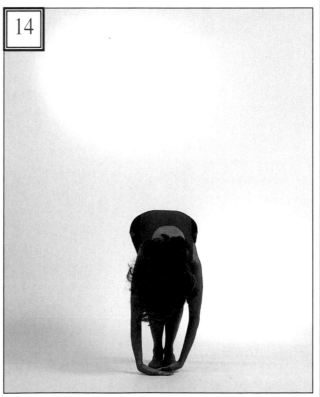

Breathing normally, relax your arms in front of you and touch the floor. Slowly straighten up and return to perfect posture.

Rise and Shine

After a long night's sleep it is very important to awaken the body slowly, avoiding any jarring movements. Muscles may have stiffened during the night, and in this condition they are prone to injuries and strains. Morning exercises should always begin by slowly easing tension with gentle stretches combined with correct breathing.

This section is really a series of warm-ups starting with movements designed to relax the muscles of the head, neck and shoulders. The Total Body Warm-up is particularly designed to loosen and relax the muscles and improve tone in the central part of the body. The easy stretching exercise that follows the Total Body Warm-up will relax tension in all the muscle groups to prepare you for the rejuvenating movements of Salute to the Sun, the last exercise in this section.

As energy levels are low in the morning, this workout is also designed to get your circulation going, to wake up and revitalize the body from top-to-toe. It is best to follow the Rise and Shine routine with exercises from Energizer or Classical.

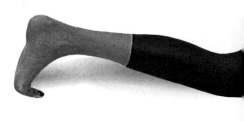

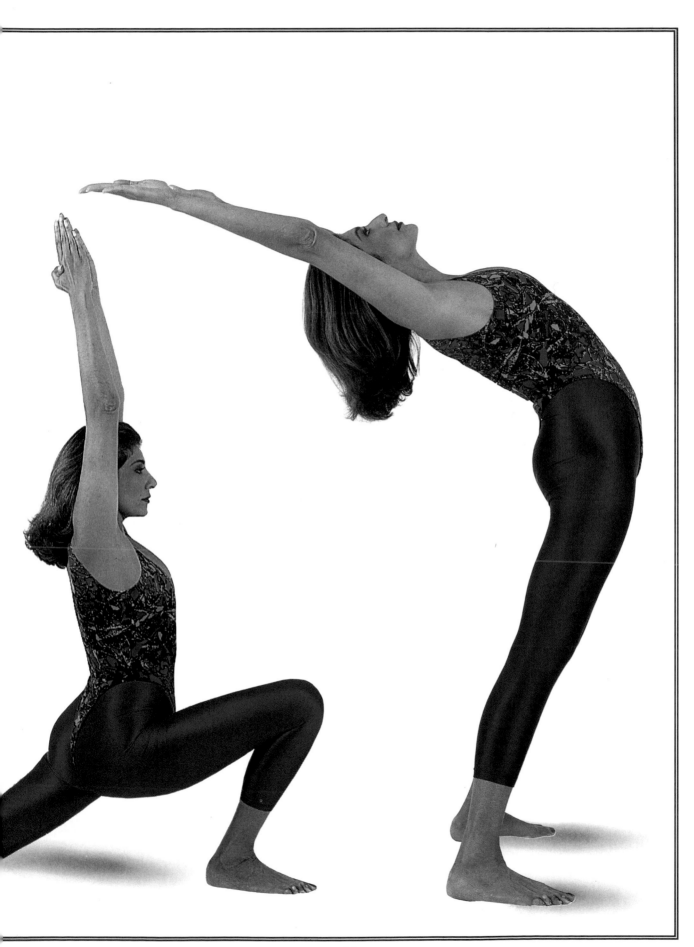

The Head Roll

The Head Roll relieves stiffness in the neck and shoulders. The exercise consists simply of rolling the head slowly in a circle without missing an inch. When the spine is not aligned properly you will experience tightness in the neck, shoulders or back. If this is the case, hold your position and breathe deeply to help the body return naturally to balance.

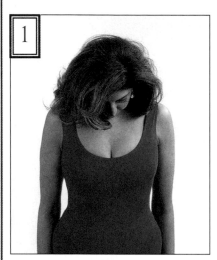

Keep your spine straight and drop your head forward, resting your chin on your chest. Breathe normally.

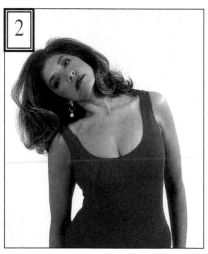

Roll your head gently up and round to the right. Try to keep your ear as close as you can to your shoulder.

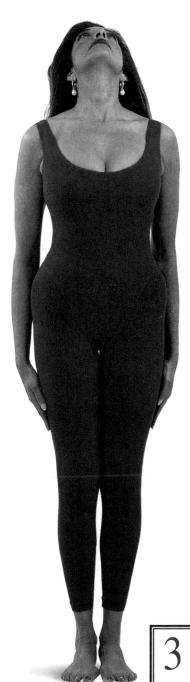

Continue the circle by rolling your head back. Relax the neck and throat and soften the face muscles, especially about the eyes.

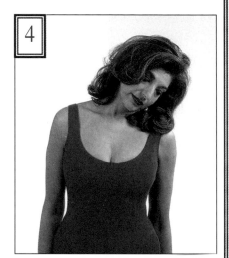

Exhale and slowly roll your head to the left. Try to keep your shoulders down to allow freedom of movement.

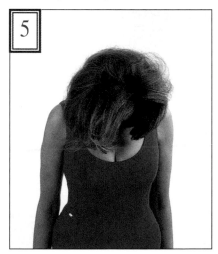

Complete the circle by rolling your head down towards your chest. Repeat the exercise in the opposite direction.

Head and Shoulders

After releasing tension in the neck with the Head Roll, move on to this exercise which includes the shoulders and relieves stiffness throughout the entire length of the spine. The Head and Shoulders exercise can be done either standing or kneeling.

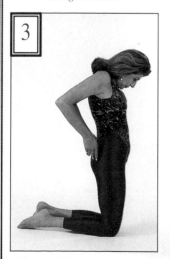

1

Kneel on the floor facing forward and inhale and exhale normally.

2

Drop your head forward to your chest, keeping your spine straight. Inhale.

3

Lift your elbows up behind you, resting your hands in the small of your back.

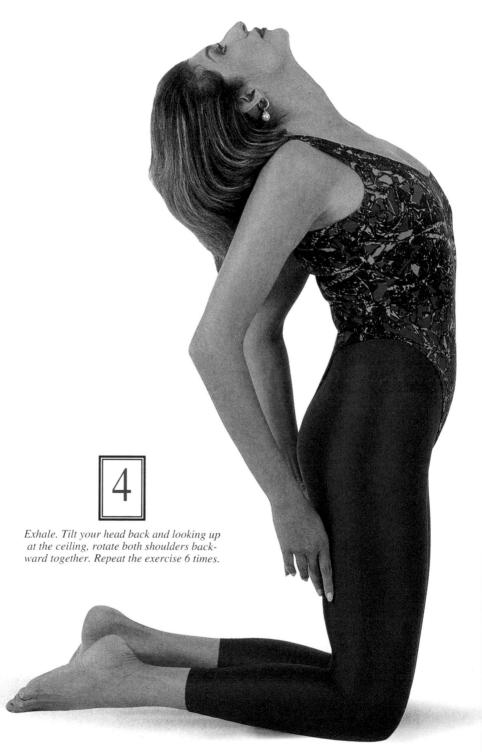

4

Exhale. Tilt your head back and looking up at the ceiling, rotate both shoulders backward together. Repeat the exercise 6 times.

Total Body Warm-up

A sedentary lifestyle and poor eating habits make many people feel lethargic. In addition, stimulants such as alcohol, caffeine and cigarettes clog up the system. The body needs help to eliminate these toxins. The Total Body Warm-up is devised to combat lethargy and cleanse the system of toxins.

This warm-up consists of ten gentle stages to awaken the body slowly, starting with movements which loosen and relax the muscles in the neck and shoulders. This sequence quickly restores energy and vitality, improving and strengthening every muscle in the central part of the body, especially the abdomen. The flexibility of the spine improves and circulation to the brain is increased. The waist, hips, abdomen, buttocks and thighs are all toned.

The stretches release tension in the muscle groups and prepare the body for the exercises that follow. As you perform the various steps, concentrate on exhaling, as this helps to relieve stiffness. Having completed the Total Body Warm-up you will feel calm, your eyes will glow and you will be filled with a sense of inner peace.

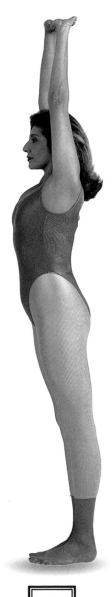

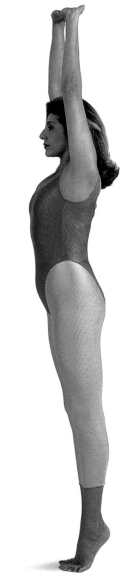

Stand tall with your feet together and your tail-bone tucked in. Inhale and raise your clasped hands above your head.

Breathing normally, balance on your toes with your eyes fixed ahead of you. Hold for 5 seconds, then return to Step 1.

RISE AND SHINE

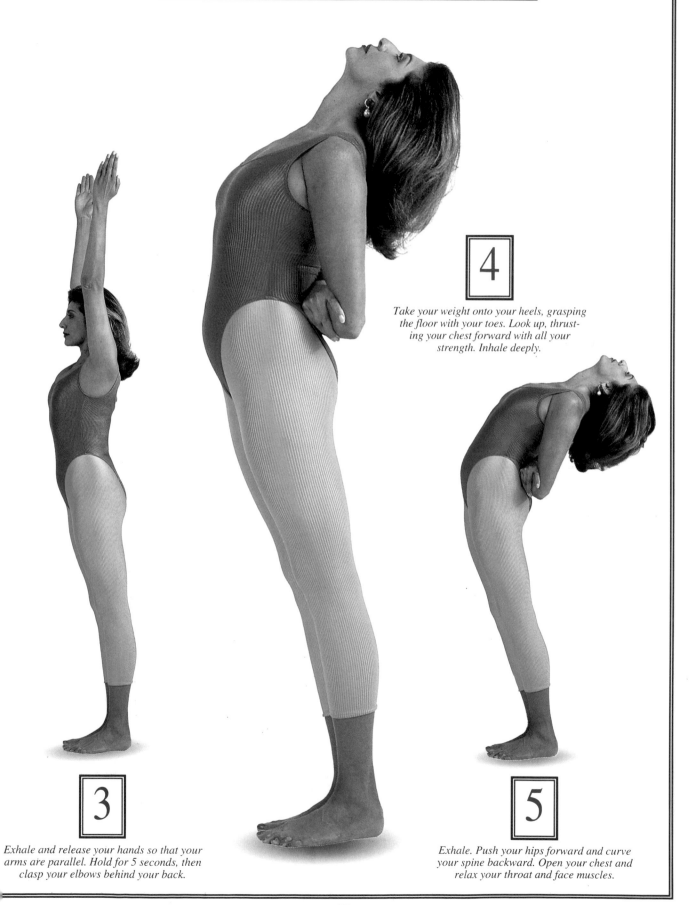

4

Take your weight onto your heels, grasping the floor with your toes. Look up, thrusting your chest forward with all your strength. Inhale deeply.

3

Exhale and release your hands so that your arms are parallel. Hold for 5 seconds, then clasp your elbows behind your back.

5

Exhale. Push your hips forward and curve your spine backward. Open your chest and relax your throat and face muscles.

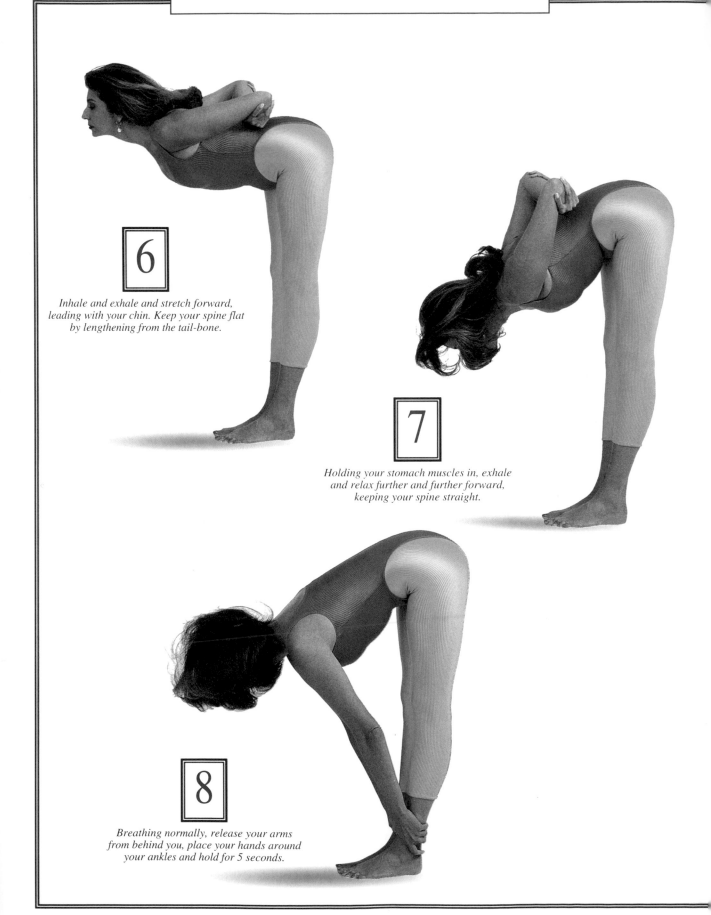

6

Inhale and exhale and stretch forward, leading with your chin. Keep your spine flat by lengthening from the tail-bone.

7

Holding your stomach muscles in, exhale and relax further and further forward, keeping your spine straight.

8

Breathing normally, release your arms from behind you, place your hands around your ankles and hold for 5 seconds.

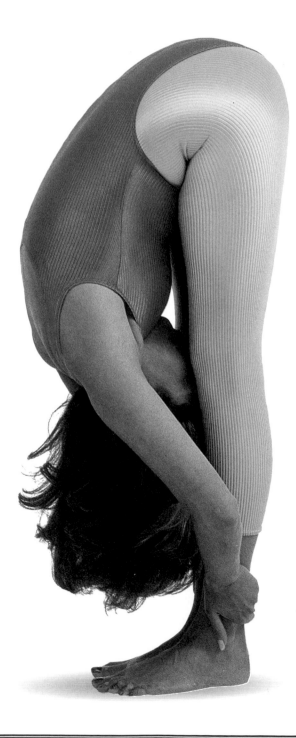

Inhale deeply then slowly exhale as you stretch forward, resting your forehead on your knees. Try to place your torso as close as possible to your thighs. Hold for 5–10 seconds.

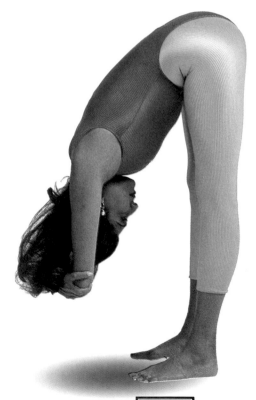

10

Part your feet to hip-width and straighten your spine from the tail-bone. Hold your elbows and stretch forward. Breathing deeply, hold for 10 seconds.

The Standing Cat Stretch

You may have seen cats and dogs stretching in a way similar to the Standing Cat Stretch. It is a marvellous stretch, with many benefits. When you are tired it restores lost energy. It strengthens the heels and ankles and gives legs a better shape. It also releases stiffness in the shoulder blades and arms and tightens the abdominal muscles, flattening the stomach. The Cat Stretch also counteracts the effects of backbends and eases any tension in the spine as it releases each part of the vertebra from the tail-bone. Placing the forehead down on the floor in Step 2 is good for soothing the nerves and relaxing deeply.

When performing this stretch, your arms might feel strained and your legs might shake a little. If this is the case, drop down to the position in Step 3 and relax. Then return to the positions in Steps 4 and 5 and hold for as long as possible. As you practice these movements, your arms and leg muscles will be gradually strengthened.

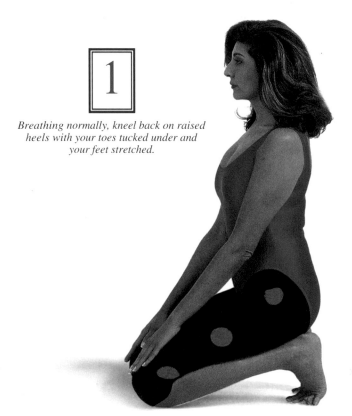

1

Breathing normally, kneel back on raised heels with your toes tucked under and your feet stretched.

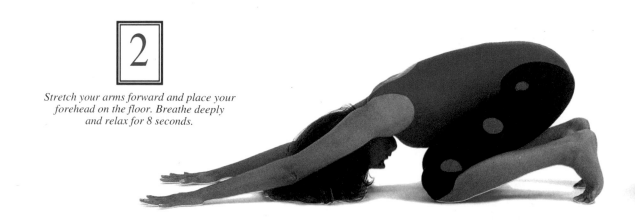

2

Stretch your arms forward and place your forehead on the floor. Breathe deeply and relax for 8 seconds.

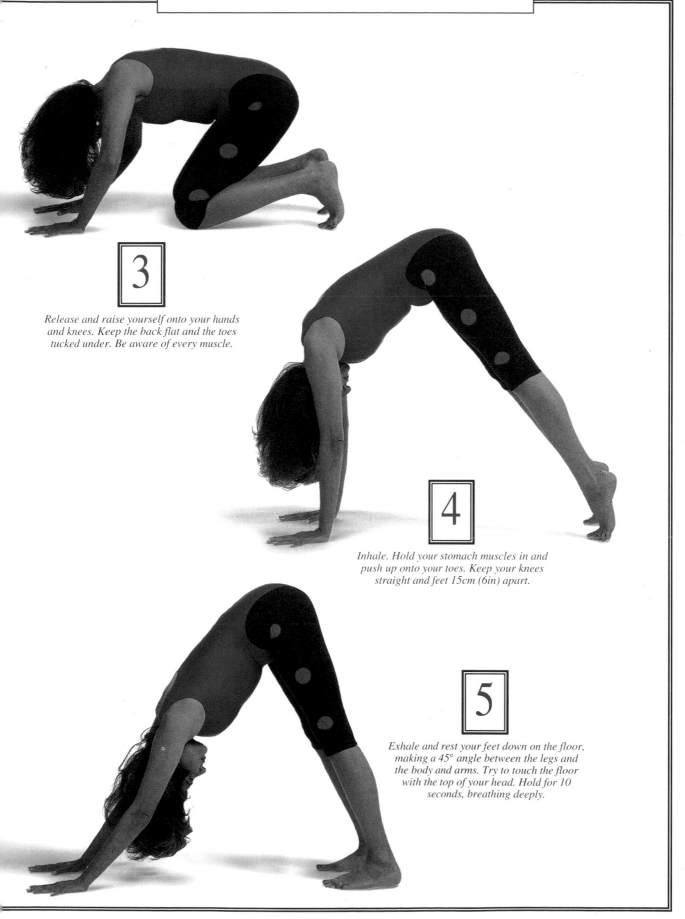

3

Release and raise yourself onto your hands and knees. Keep the back flat and the toes tucked under. Be aware of every muscle.

4

Inhale. Hold your stomach muscles in and push up onto your toes. Keep your knees straight and feet 15cm (6in) apart.

5

Exhale and rest your feet down on the floor, making a 45° angle between the legs and the body and arms. Try to touch the floor with the top of your head. Hold for 10 seconds, breathing deeply.

Salute to the Sun

Salute to the Sun is a traditional Yoga warm-up, which has a wonderful, rejuvenating effect. The slow, gentle movements exercise and tone every muscle in the body and improve the body's flexibility, stamina, poise and suppleness. When performing Salute to the Sun, keep the energy flowing as you move from one position to another. Pay particular attention to your breathing pattern, as it is most important for increasing energy levels and vitality. Once you have managed to build up your stamina, you should aim to perform the whole sequence ten times on each side.

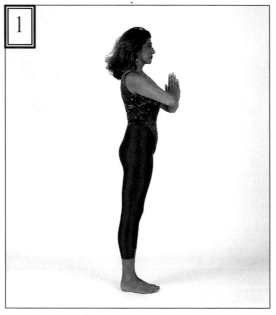

Breathe normally. Looking ahead, stand tall in perfect posture with palms together and shoulders down.

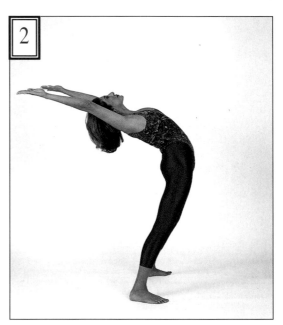

Inhale and step to the right. Fling your arms over your head and reach back behind you.

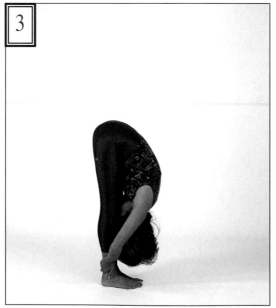

Exhale as you bring your feet together and relax down. Clasp the ankles and try to touch your knees with your forehead. Bend your knees slightly, if you wish.

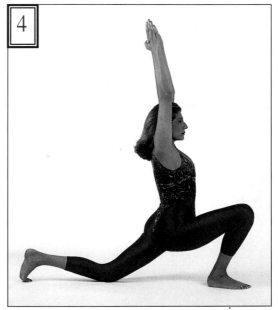

Inhale and take the left leg back as far as you can with the toes tucked under, then flatten the leg as in Step 11. Raise your arms, with palms together. Breathe normally.

As with all the Rise and Shine exercises, Salute to the Sun should be performed with a graceful flow of energy. As you familiarize yourself with the sequence, you will eventually be able to move from one position to the next with confidence and fluidity – like an accomplished dancer.

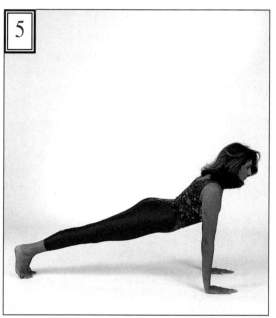

Extend both legs behind you and raise yourself onto your hands and feet, keeping your arms straight.

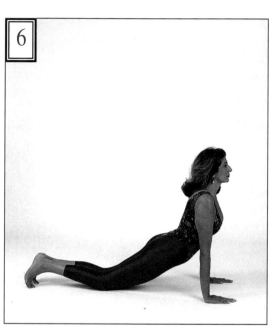

Drop to your knees and keep your gaze straight ahead. Try not to make any unnecessary movements.

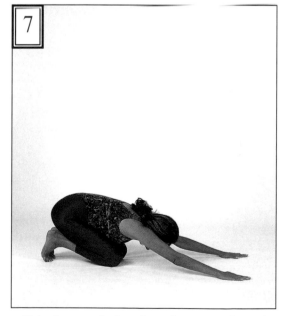

Sit back on your heels and stretch your arms forward to release your spine.

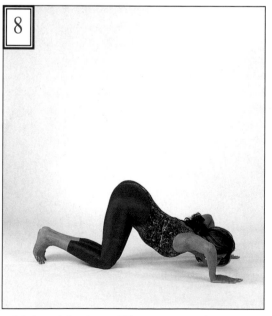

Inhale and dive forward like a serpent, with your chin sliding close to the floor. Bend your elbows.

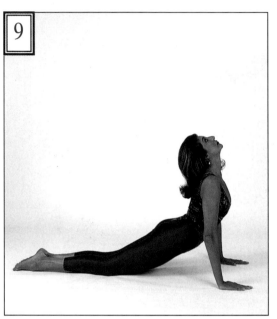

Still inhaling, straighten your arms and swing forward
with your hips and curve your spine, looking up.

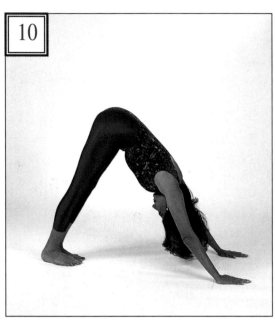

Exhale, raise your hips, and drop your toes and heels
down onto the floor, stretching the entire spine.

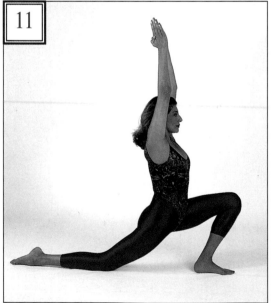

Inhale and bring your left leg forward, extending your
right leg back (as for left leg in Step 4). Raise your
arms, with palms together. Breathe normally.

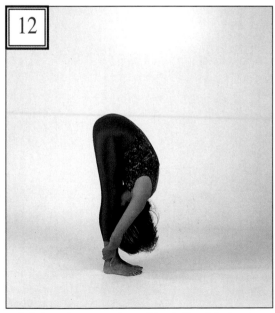

Exhale and return to the position in Step 3 by leaning
forward and bringing your right foot to join the left,
clasping the ankles, then straightening the knees.

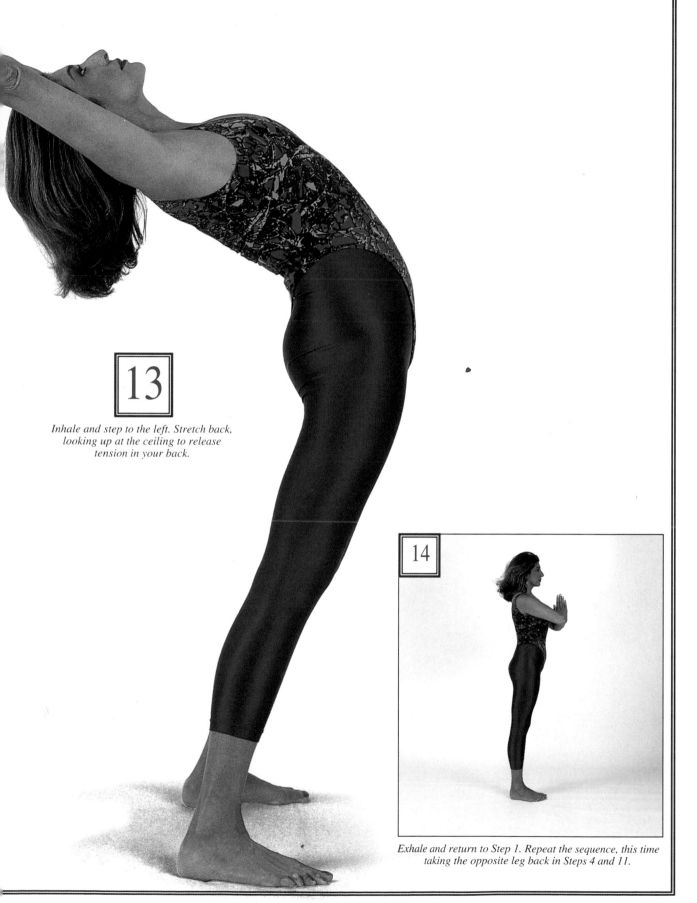

13

Inhale and step to the left. Stretch back, looking up at the ceiling to release tension in your back.

14

Exhale and return to Step 1. Repeat the sequence, this time taking the opposite leg back in Steps 4 and 11.

Energizer

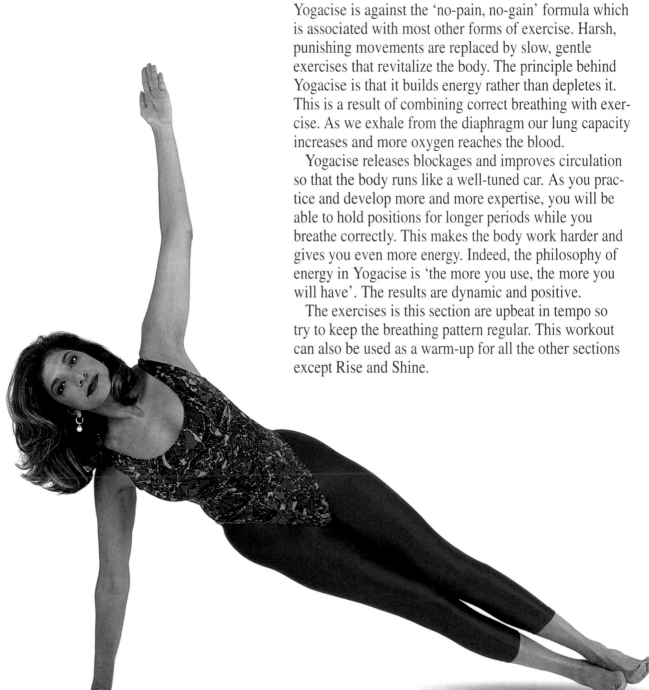

Yogacise is against the 'no-pain, no-gain' formula which is associated with most other forms of exercise. Harsh, punishing movements are replaced by slow, gentle exercises that revitalize the body. The principle behind Yogacise is that it builds energy rather than depletes it. This is a result of combining correct breathing with exercise. As we exhale from the diaphragm our lung capacity increases and more oxygen reaches the blood.

Yogacise releases blockages and improves circulation so that the body runs like a well-tuned car. As you practice and develop more and more expertise, you will be able to hold positions for longer periods while you breathe correctly. This makes the body work harder and gives you even more energy. Indeed, the philosophy of energy in Yogacise is 'the more you use, the more you will have'. The results are dynamic and positive.

The exercises is this section are upbeat in tempo so try to keep the breathing pattern regular. This workout can also be used as a warm-up for all the other sections except Rise and Shine.

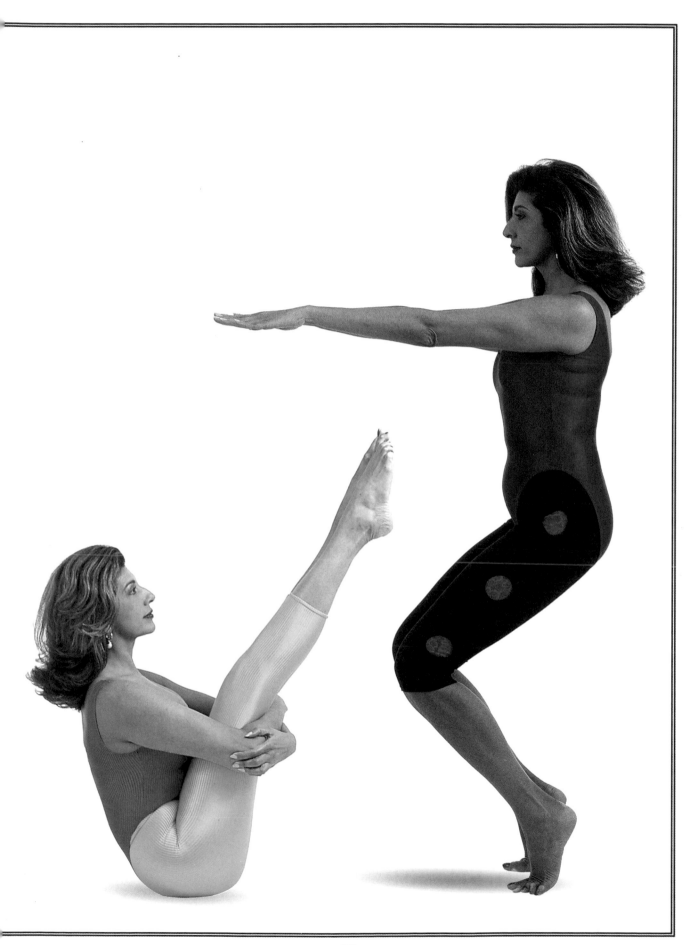

The Jump

The Jump is a wonderful exercise that energizes and rejuvenates the entire body. Jumping increases the heartbeat and circulation, leaving you with a feeling of youth and vitality. Because this exercise is fairly strenuous, it is important to keep your breathing regular. Remember to always breathe through the nose.

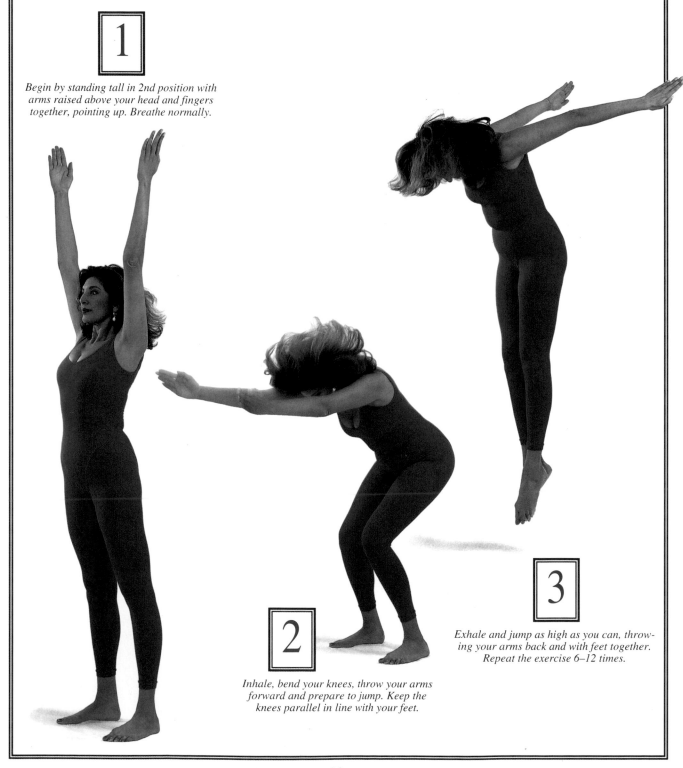

1

Begin by standing tall in 2nd position with arms raised above your head and fingers together, pointing up. Breathe normally.

2

Inhale, bend your knees, throw your arms forward and prepare to jump. Keep the knees parallel in line with your feet.

3

Exhale and jump as high as you can, throwing your arms back and with feet together. Repeat the exercise 6–12 times.

Energy Boost

This exercise is more advanced because it combines jumps with lunges. Coordination is very important and it is useful to visualize yourself in the finished pose before you begin. The movements should be graceful with a continuous flow between one position and another. Your pulse rate will increase immediately, giving you an extra energy boost.

Stand tall with your elbows raised just above shoulder level, your feet together and knees bent.

Inhale and prepare to jump by standing on your toes with your arms down by your sides and slightly back.

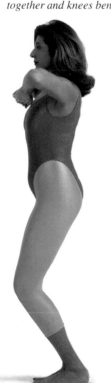

Jump as high as you can, throwing your arms above your head and kicking your right leg back.

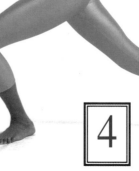

Exhale and finish with the right leg extended, the left knee bent and left heel down. Repeat 6–12 times, reversing legs.

Knee Bend 1

The Knee Bend strengthens the lower spine and the muscles in the legs, thighs, calves, hips and upper arms. It improves circulation and helps to relieve ailments such as rheumatism and arthritis in the legs.

These exercises employ 'grounding' techniques and by learning determination and patience you will find everyday problems easier to cope with.

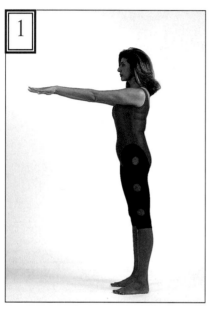

1

Stand tall in perfect posture and raise your arms to shoulder height. Focus on one spot in front of you.

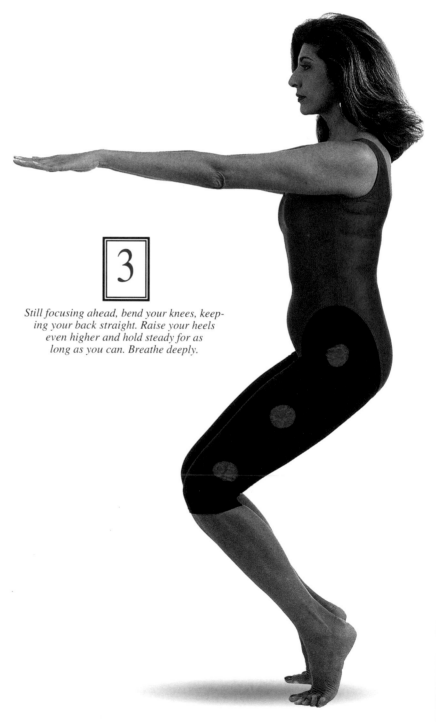

3

Still focusing ahead, bend your knees, keeping your back straight. Raise your heels even higher and hold steady for as long as you can. Breathe deeply.

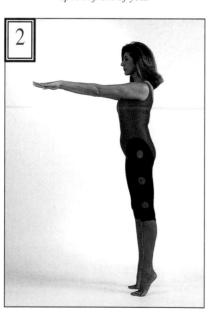

2

Balance high on your toes, without rocking forward or back. Make sure your little toe is pushed down onto the floor.

Knee Bend 2

This exercise expands your breathing capacity and so energizes the body. It helps to relieve sciatica by strengthening the discs in the lumbar region of the spine and the final hanging position is good for soothing the nerves. A lot of strength is needed in Step 2 – you may find it easier if you imagine there is a chair behind you, and then take your tail-bone back as if to sit on it.

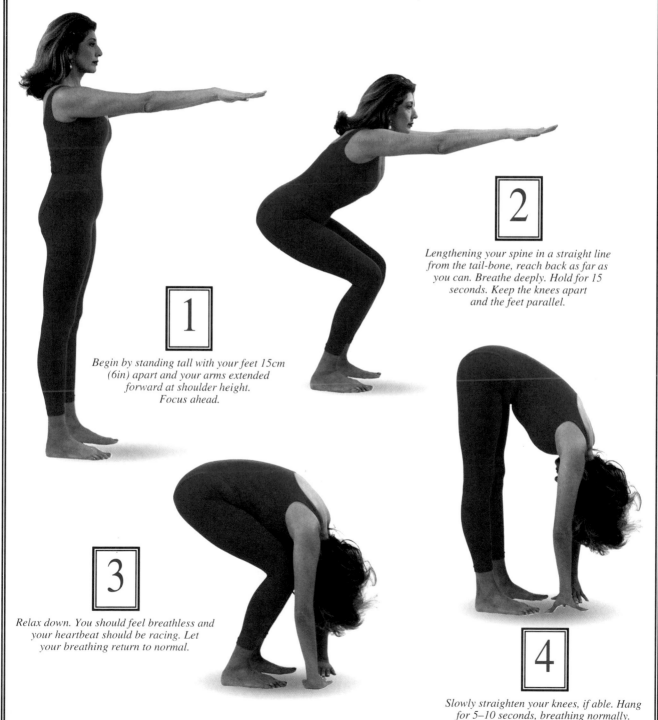

1

Begin by standing tall with your feet 15cm (6in) apart and your arms extended forward at shoulder height. Focus ahead.

2

Lengthening your spine in a straight line from the tail-bone, reach back as far as you can. Breathe deeply. Hold for 15 seconds. Keep the knees apart and the feet parallel.

3

Relax down. You should feel breathless and your heartbeat should be racing. Let your breathing return to normal.

4

Slowly straighten your knees, if able. Hang for 5–10 seconds, breathing normally. Inhale and gently return to Step 1.

Knee Bend 3

This is a vigorous exercise, requiring a lot of strength and stamina, so do not attempt it until you have mastered Knee Bends 1 and 2. You may experience quivering in your thighs, which indicates weak muscles. This knee bend helps to reduce cellulite, increases circulation in the legs and is great preparation for skiing or water-skiing.

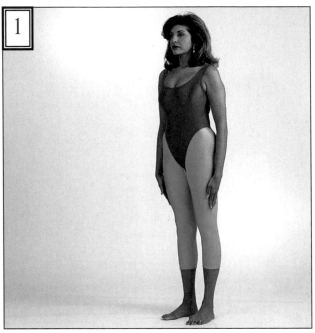

Stand in 2nd position, with feet 15cm (6in) apart and arms down by your sides. Focus on a point straight ahead of you.

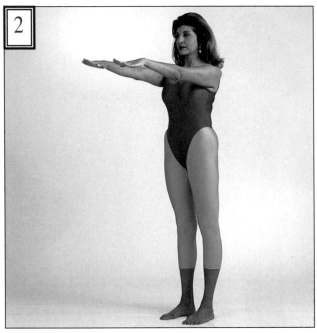

Raise your arms to shoulder height. Tighten your stomach and buttock muscles and raise the muscle above the kneecaps.

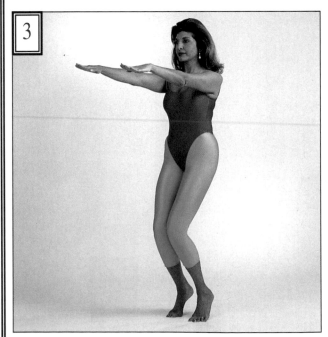

Knock your knees together and raise your heels off the floor. Balance without rocking and hold for 5 seconds.

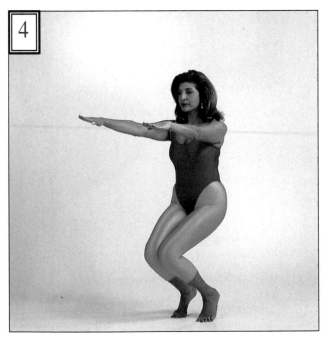

Keeping the spine straight, bend your knees and continue to focus straight ahead. Nothing should move but the knees.

5

Reaching a 90° angle with the hips and knees, breathe deeply and hold all the muscles tight for as long as you can.

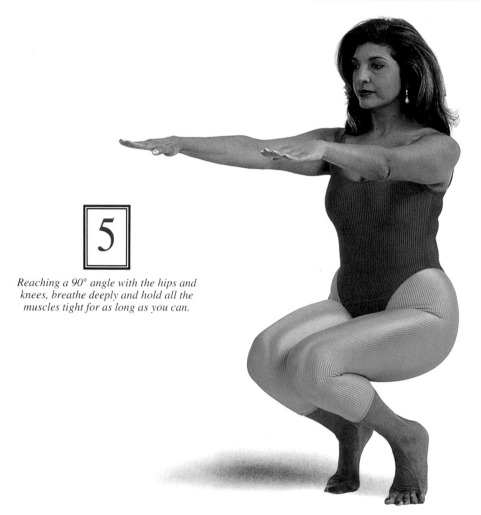

6

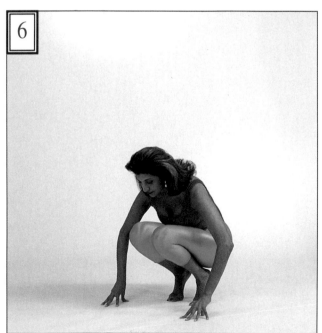

Relax down and wait for your breathing to return to normal. Energy should be flowing swiftly through the body.

7

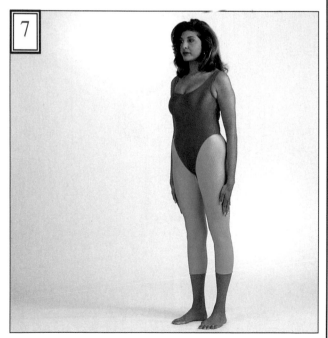

Slowly uncurl the spine and return to Step 1. Center yourself and hold for 5 seconds.

The Tree

Balance comes from a focused mind. Although this exercise may look very simple, unless you concentrate hard you will be unable to keep still. Think of yourself as a statue. The leg you stand on must remain straight. Grip the floor with your toes and lift the knee upward by tensing the muscle above the kneecap. Be very careful not to strain yourself.

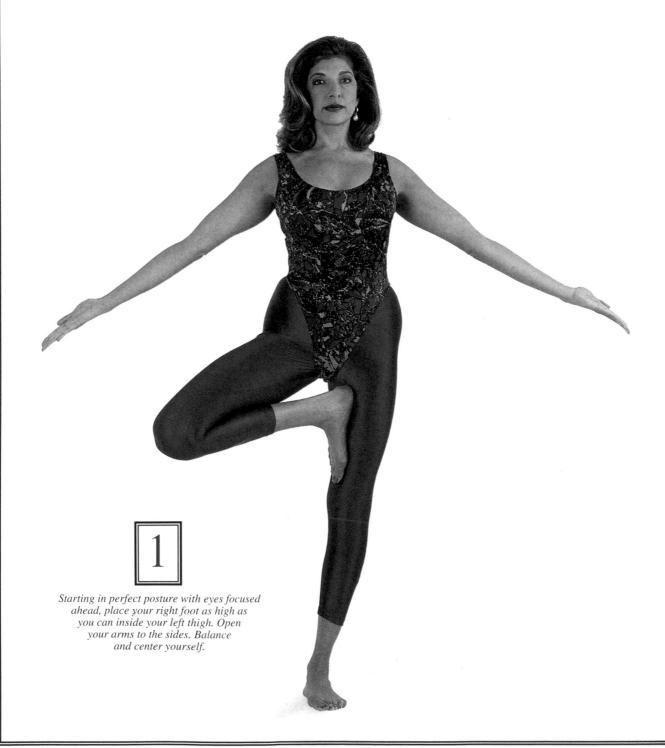

1

Starting in perfect posture with eyes focused ahead, place your right foot as high as you can inside your left thigh. Open your arms to the sides. Balance and center yourself.

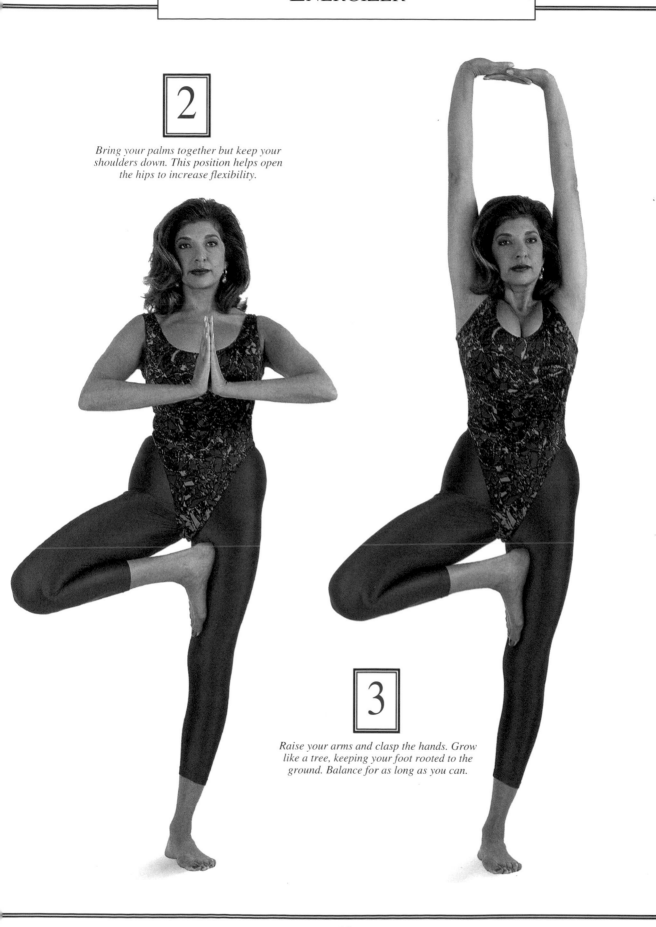

2

Bring your palms together but keep your shoulders down. This position helps open the hips to increase flexibility.

3

Raise your arms and clasp the hands. Grow like a tree, keeping your foot rooted to the ground. Balance for as long as you can.

The Letter T

This is the only Yogacise pose that should be held for no longer than 10 seconds. It is a powerful, dynamic stretch that increases the pulse rate and the heartbeat, strengthens the heart muscles and increases lung capacity. The increased circulation it produces will energize the whole body.

The Letter T teaches you perfect body control and improves your mental powers. It not only firms hips,

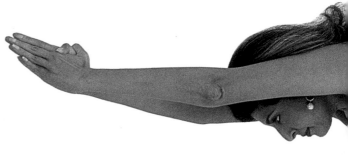

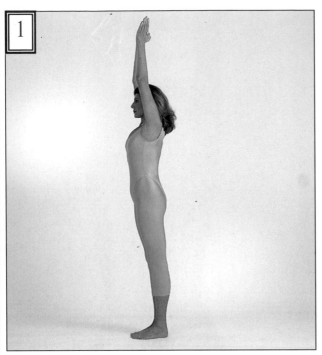

1

Stand tall with feet together and stretch your arms over your head, close to the ears. Press your palms together and cross thumbs.

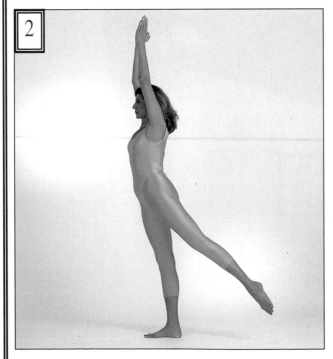

2

Point your left leg behind you keeping your knee straight. Focus on one spot ahead of you.

buttocks and upper thighs but also improves muscle tone in the shoulders and upper arms because of the position of the outstretched arms with straight elbows.

As you bend forward, continue to think that you are stretching upward. This will stop you curving your back. Once you have reached Step 3, continue to stretch with all your strength.

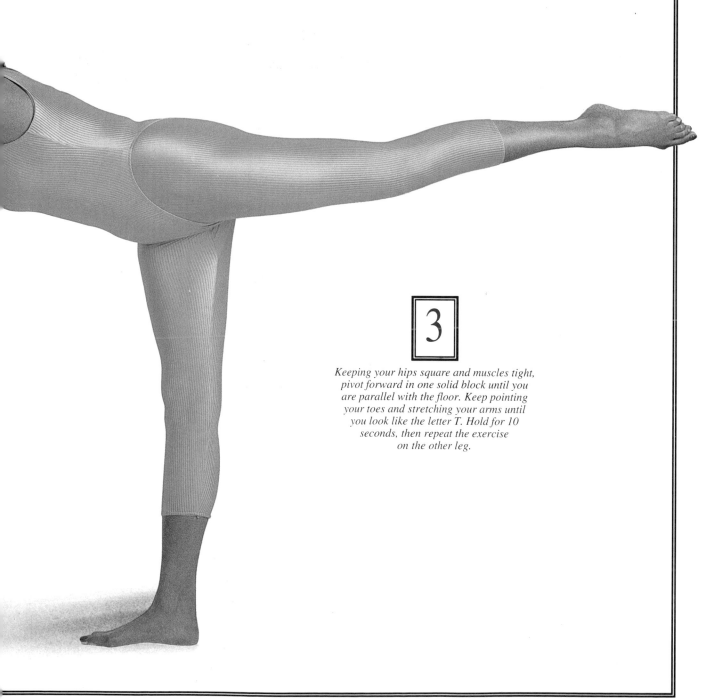

3

Keeping your hips square and muscles tight, pivot forward in one solid block until you are parallel with the floor. Keep pointing your toes and stretching your arms until you look like the letter T. Hold for 10 seconds, then repeat the exercise on the other leg.

The Leg Lift

These leg lifts strengthen the abdominal muscles and increase flexibility in the hips and hamstrings. They also improve your concentration by encouraging you to focus on your breathing. As you change positions, keep the movements precise and your mind and body as still as possible. If you find it difficult to bring your head to your knee, do not force it. Eventually your hamstrings will loosen to increase the suppleness of your legs.

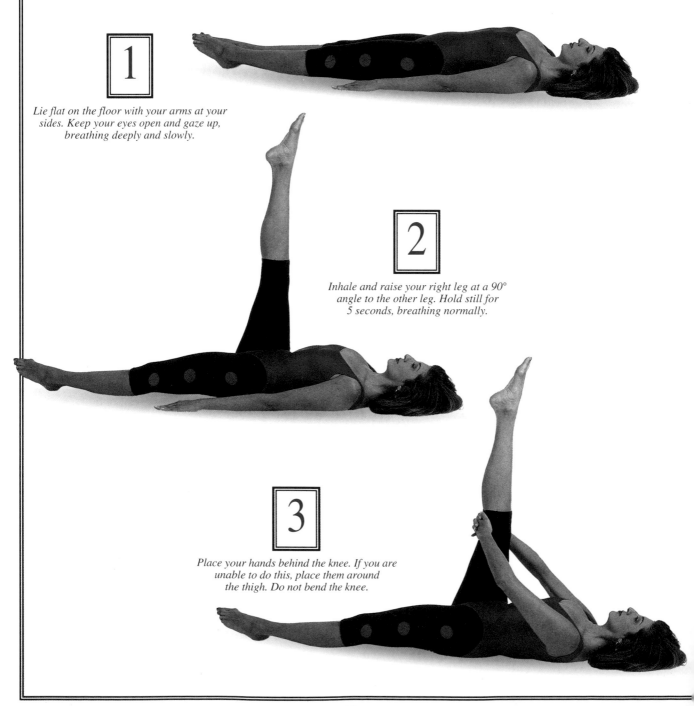

1 *Lie flat on the floor with your arms at your sides. Keep your eyes open and gaze up, breathing deeply and slowly.*

2 *Inhale and raise your right leg at a 90° angle to the other leg. Hold still for 5 seconds, breathing normally.*

3 *Place your hands behind the knee. If you are unable to do this, place them around the thigh. Do not bend the knee.*

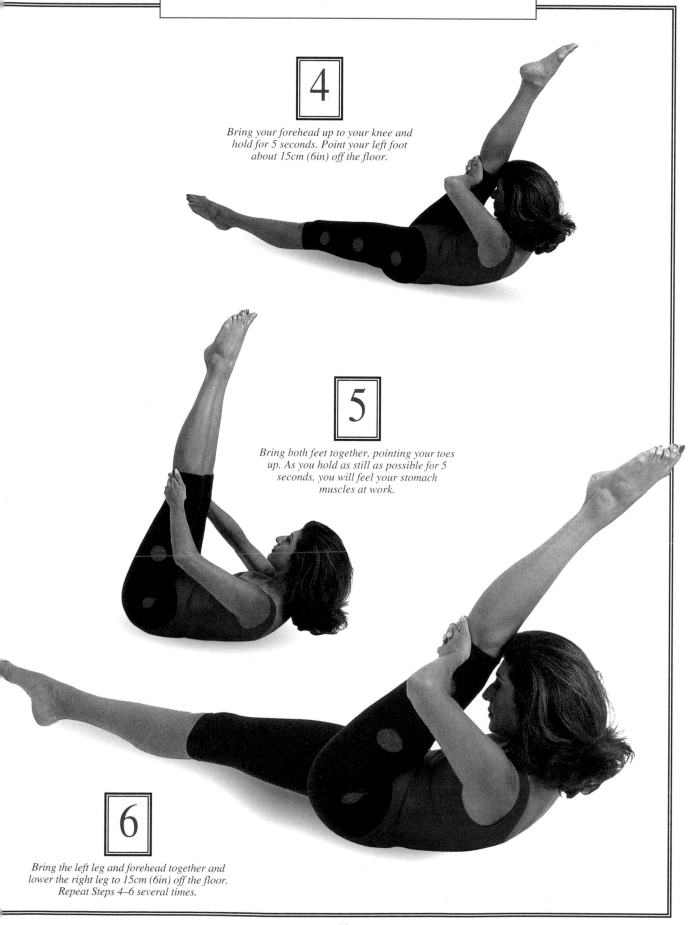

4

Bring your forehead up to your knee and hold for 5 seconds. Point your left foot about 15cm (6in) off the floor.

5

Bring both feet together, pointing your toes up. As you hold as still as possible for 5 seconds, you will feel your stomach muscles at work.

6

Bring the left leg and forehead together and lower the right leg to 15cm (6in) off the floor. Repeat Steps 4–6 several times.

The Back Leg Lift

The Back Leg Lift is a particularly good exercise for the buttock muscles. As people grow older their buttock muscles start to sag and they find that the backside is a very difficult area to isolate and tone. Most Yogacise exercises firm these muscles because of the constant attention to posture – the tail-bone is always tucked in and the buttocks are held tight. The Back Leg Lift also strengthens the lower back and tones the abdominal and leg muscles. It also helps to cure ailments such as sciatica and lumbago. This is a strenuous exercise, so make sure you keep your breathing deep and even throughout.

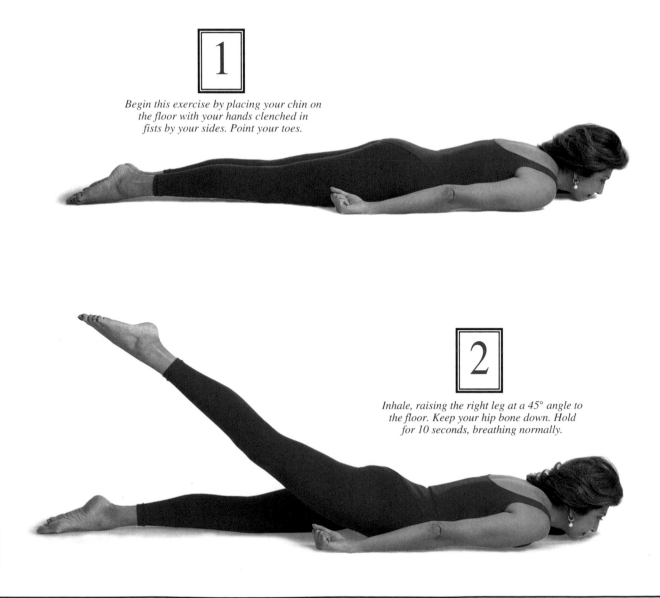

1

Begin this exercise by placing your chin on the floor with your hands clenched in fists by your sides. Point your toes.

2

Inhale, raising the right leg at a 45° angle to the floor. Keep your hip bone down. Hold for 10 seconds, breathing normally.

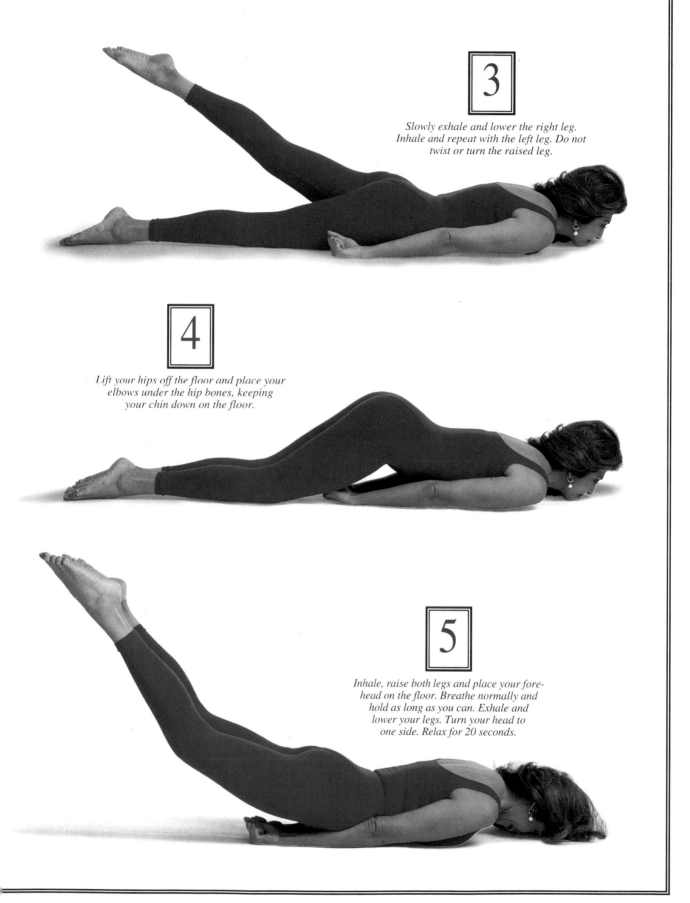

3

Slowly exhale and lower the right leg. Inhale and repeat with the left leg. Do not twist or turn the raised leg.

4

Lift your hips off the floor and place your elbows under the hip bones, keeping your chin down on the floor.

5

Inhale, raise both legs and place your forehead on the floor. Breathe normally and hold as long as you can. Exhale and lower your legs. Turn your head to one side. Relax for 20 seconds.

The Jet

The Jet is a fast-paced exercise that will increase your pulse rate, improve overall flexibility and build up your stamina. It strengthens the lower back and improves the muscle tone of the hips, buttocks and thighs. In addition, balancing on your hip bone tightens the abdominal muscles. By Step 5, you will feel like a jet plane ready for take-off.

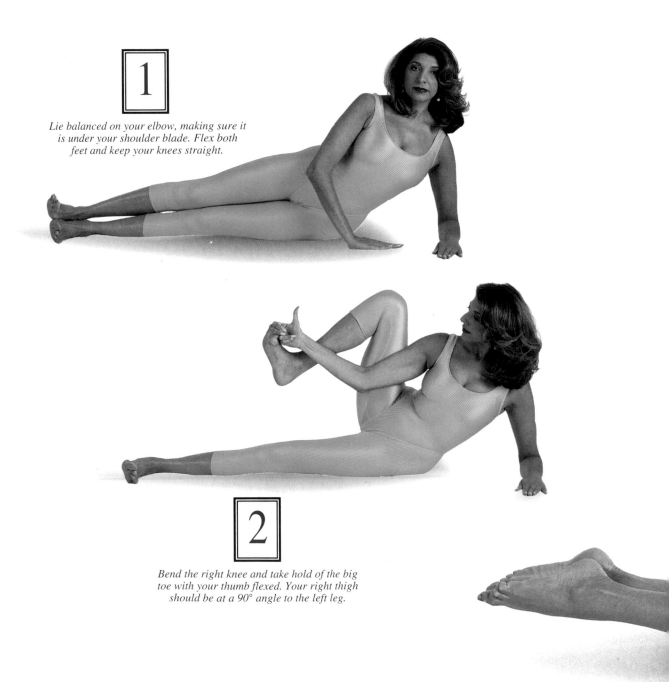

1

Lie balanced on your elbow, making sure it is under your shoulder blade. Flex both feet and keep your knees straight.

2

Bend the right knee and take hold of the big toe with your thumb flexed. Your right thigh should be at a 90° angle to the left leg.

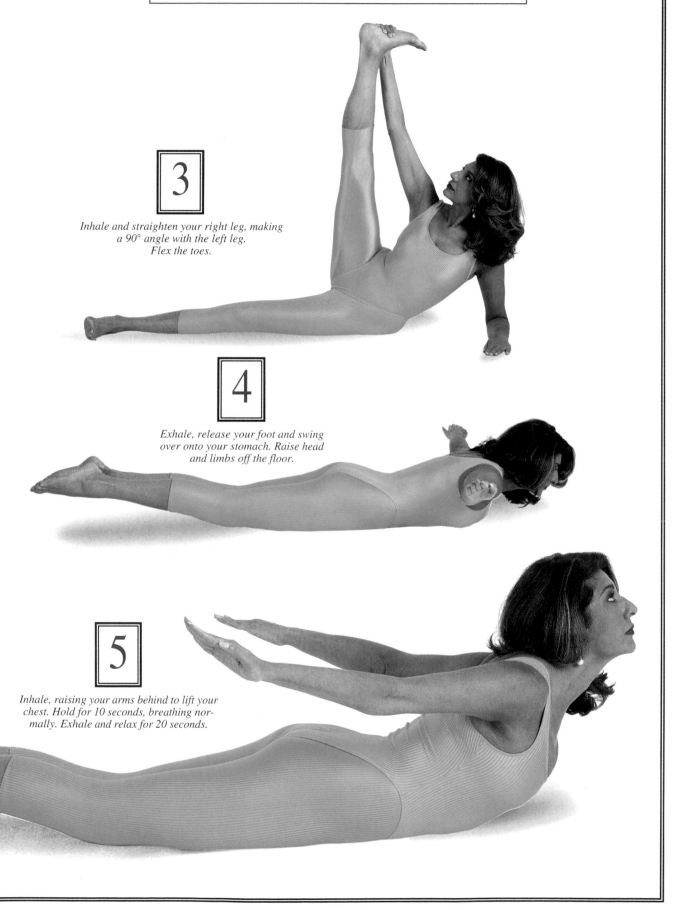

3

Inhale and straighten your right leg, making a 90° angle with the left leg. Flex the toes.

4

Exhale, release your foot and swing over onto your stomach. Raise head and limbs off the floor.

5

Inhale, raising your arms behind to lift your chest. Hold for 10 seconds, breathing normally. Exhale and relax for 20 seconds.

The Sitting Balance

This exercise strengthens the lower back and tones the abdominal muscles. It is particularly good for flattening the stomach, especially after having a baby. It is more difficult to balance whilst in a sitting position because you have to keep your spine straight as well as supporting your weight without using your leg muscles. On completing the exercise, relax down on your back into Step 1 of Deep Relaxation (see page 125).

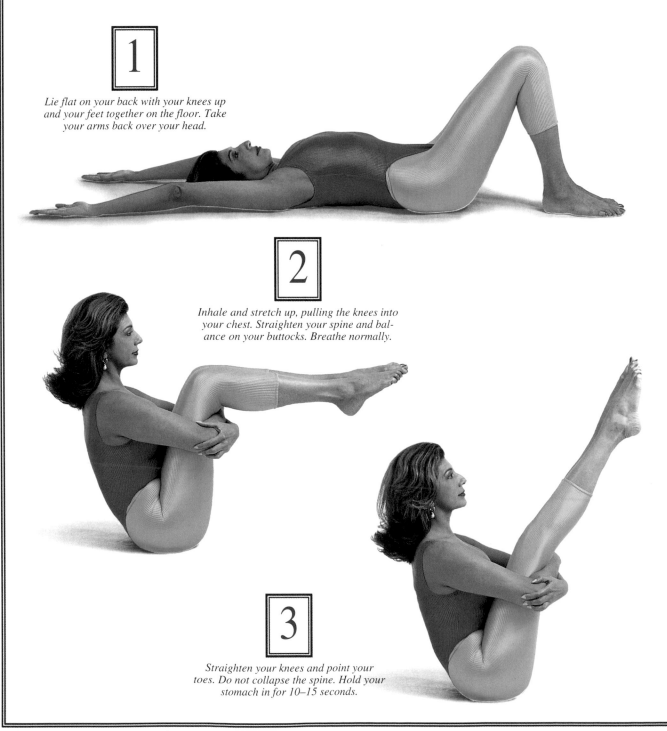

1

Lie flat on your back with your knees up and your feet together on the floor. Take your arms back over your head.

2

Inhale and stretch up, pulling the knees into your chest. Straighten your spine and balance on your buttocks. Breathe normally.

3

Straighten your knees and point your toes. Do not collapse the spine. Hold your stomach in for 10–15 seconds.

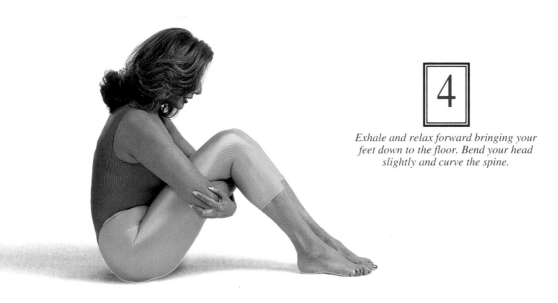

4

Exhale and relax forward bringing your feet down to the floor. Bend your head slightly and curve the spine.

5

Stretch your legs out and lengthen from the tail-bone. Breathe normally and extend your chin forward. Put your fingers round your big toes and flex the thumbs.

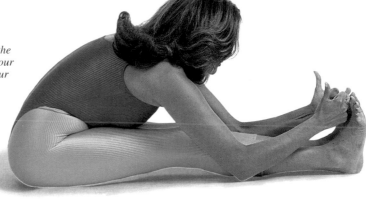

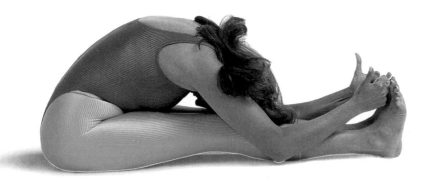

6

Extend forward as far as you can, then drop your forehead to your knees for 20 seconds. To release, sit tall and relax back.

One-Arm Balance

The One-Arm Balance is excellent for strengthening the forearms, upper arms and shoulders. Although it may look difficult, when your body is in perfect alignment, you will be surprised at how easy it is to perform. If the shoulders, hips and feet are in a straight line, your body becomes weightless and you will find that you are in total control.

A great deal of energy is required for the balancing positions because of the increased concentration they demand. As the positions become more challenging, breathe deeply into the movement and you will find that your energy levels increase.

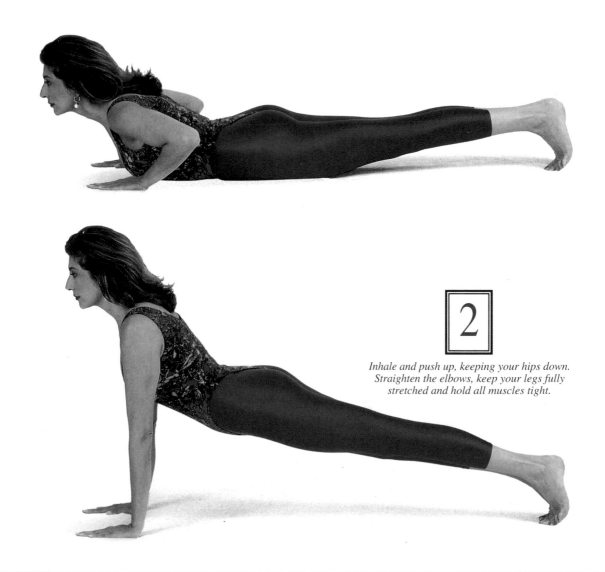

1

Lie on your stomach with your spine straight, toes tucked under and hands below your shoulder blades. Look ahead.

2

Inhale and push up, keeping your hips down. Straighten the elbows, keep your legs fully stretched and hold all muscles tight.

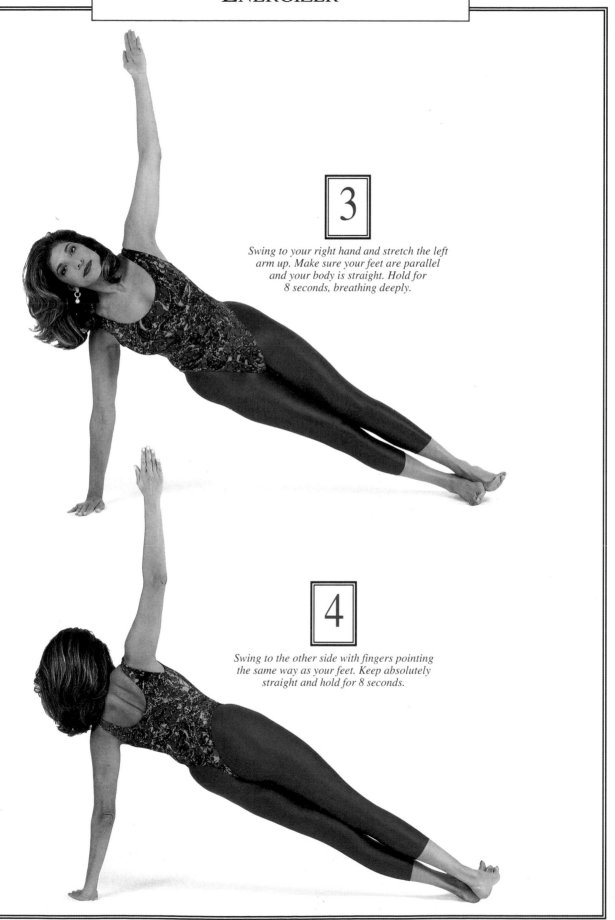

3

Swing to your right hand and stretch the left arm up. Make sure your feet are parallel and your body is straight. Hold for 8 seconds, breathing deeply.

4

Swing to the other side with fingers pointing the same way as your feet. Keep absolutely straight and hold for 8 seconds.

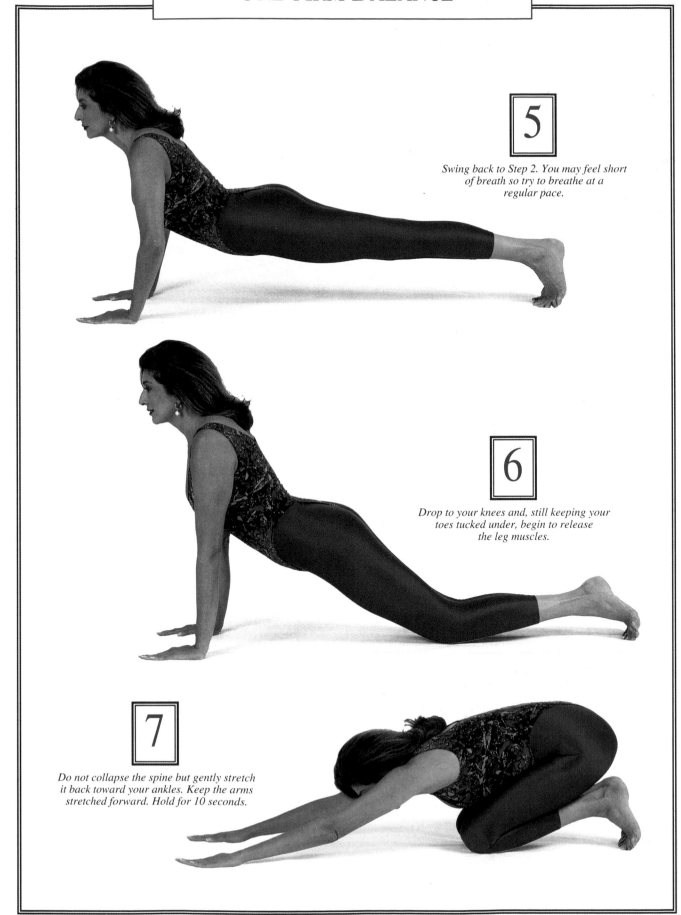

5

Swing back to Step 2. You may feel short of breath so try to breathe at a regular pace.

6

Drop to your knees and, still keeping your toes tucked under, begin to release the leg muscles.

7

Do not collapse the spine but gently stretch it back toward your ankles. Keep the arms stretched forward. Hold for 10 seconds.

The Stretch With Hands

Many people will be discouraged when they first try this exercise because it looks simple but is actually quite challenging. You may find that you can do it on one side but not the other. With regular practice, however, you will feel tense muscles loosen. Since this stretch is designed to increase chest capacity and release tension in the neck and shoulders, it is important to keep your shoulders square so that the upper back stays in line.

3

Repeat the exercise on the other side, taking your right arm behind you and your left arm over your shoulder.

1

Sitting on your heels with a straight spine, take your left arm behind your lower back. Make sure your palm is facing up. Bend the right elbow and raise the arm overhead.

2

Move your left hand up the spine as close to the shoulder blades as possible and try to clasp your fingertips for 8 seconds.

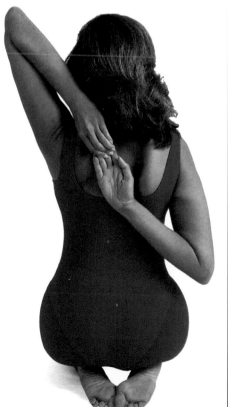

Breathing With Arms

Most people breathe using only 10 per cent of their lung capacity. This leads to lethargy and a depletion of energy and aggravates breathing problems such as asthma, emphysema and shortness of breath.

This breathing technique is designed to combat these problems. It expands the lung capacity and improves circulation throughout the body. As you inhale deeply and slowly through the nose, you will feel your lungs fill with air. When your elbows are lifted, hold your breath for a few seconds and feel the tension in your neck, shoulders and elbows. Then as you exhale though your mouth, let the air escape slowly and steadily.

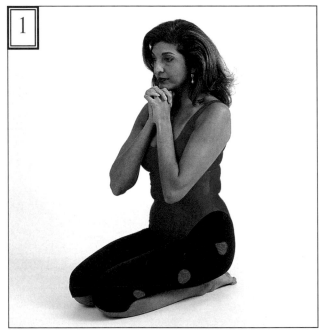

Sit on your heels with hands clasped under your chin. Make sure you keep your chin parallel to the ground.

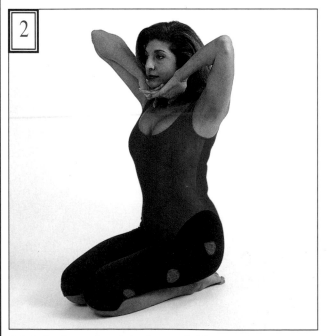

Inhale for 6 seconds and simultaneously lift your elbows up as high as possible. Do not bend forward. Keep your spine straight.

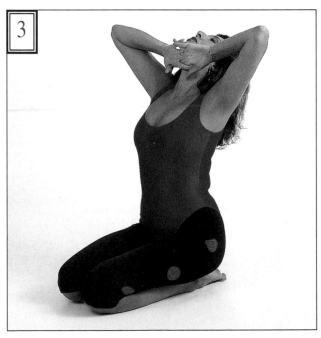

Keeping the movements fluid, slowly exhale through your mouth as you look upward and drop your head backward.

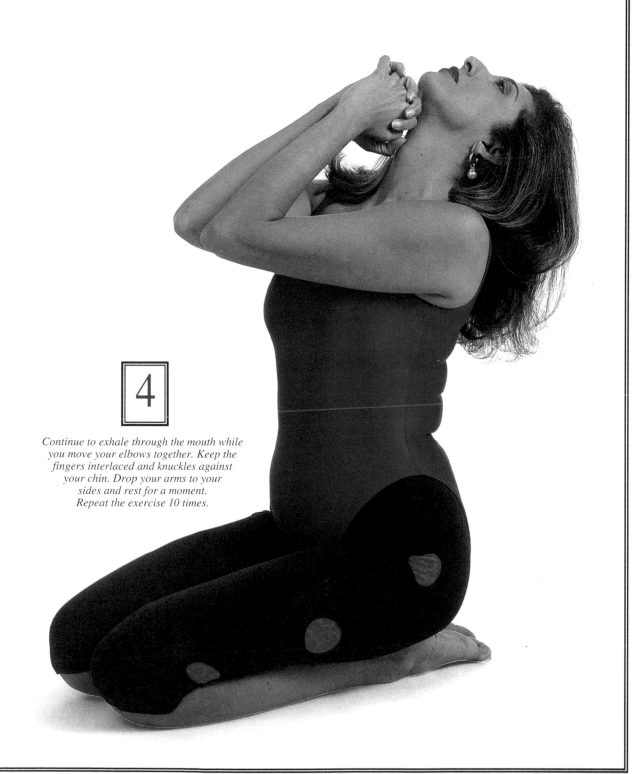

4

Continue to exhale through the mouth while you move your elbows together. Keep the fingers interlaced and knuckles against your chin. Drop your arms to your sides and rest for a moment. Repeat the exercise 10 times.

Ultimate Stretch

Stretching is the very best way to achieve overall top-to-toe fitness. In Yogacise the muscles are stretched lengthways to their maximum. This elongation improves their tone and eliminates the fat around each cell, helping to reduce cellulite and improve body shape.

Stretching affects the health of the whole body by improving blood circulation and calming and soothing the nervous system. It is the gentlest way to release tension in the muscle groups, and the forward, sideways and backward movements allow the body

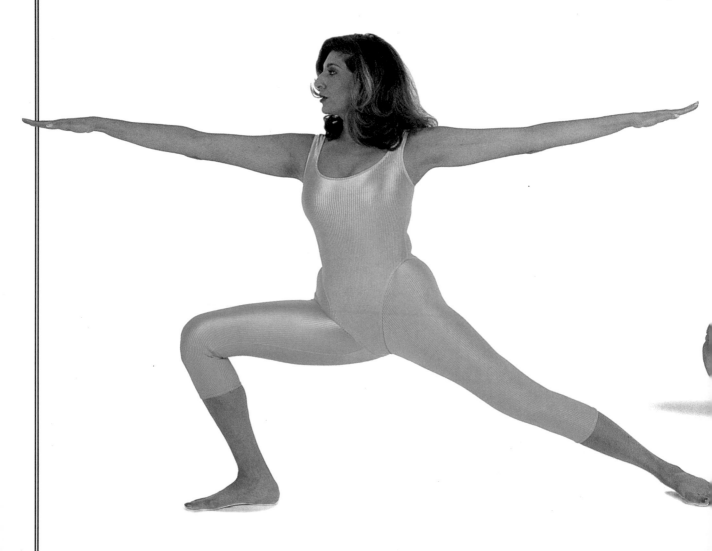

to return to perfect alignment. Stretching increases flexibility and suppleness. It also helps to detoxify the body, stimulates lymphatic drainage and strengthens the immune system, helping to prevent common ailments.

As you stretch in this workout, think of yourself as a rubber band. Keep pulling and stretching with all your physical strength. On completion, you will feel an intense release of energy – like releasing a rubber band that has been stretched to its limit.

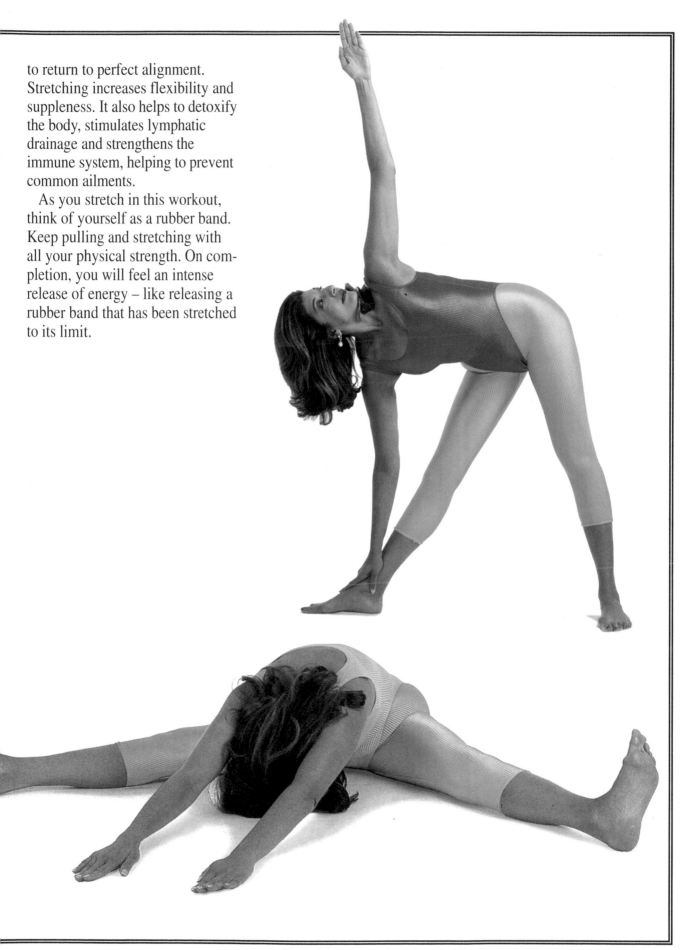

Stretch Up 1

Stretching up corrects bad posture and bestows grace and equilibrium. Plant your feet firmly on the ground and grow upward by lifting the muscles above the kneecaps, and the muscles of the thighs, hips and waist. Lift your chest but push your shoulder blades down. Stretch your neck but keep your chin level as if a string were pulling you up from the top of your head.

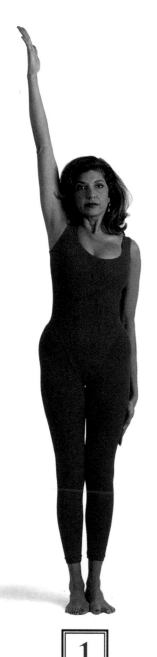

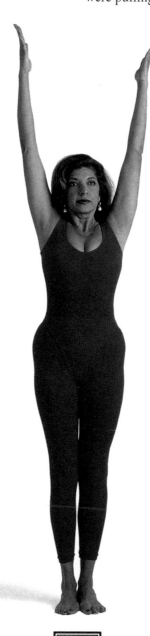

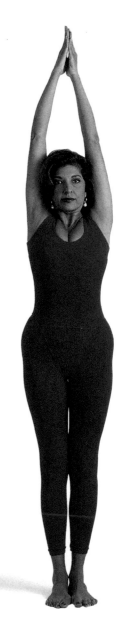

1

Stand tall in perfect posture, and distribute your weight evenly between your heels and toes. Raise your right arm.

2

Grasp the floor with your toes and raise your left arm. Stretch up, keeping the shoulders down. Hold for 5 seconds.

3

Bring your palms together, keeping your elbows straight and as close to your ears as possible. Hold for 5 seconds.

Stretch Up 2

This stretch takes you one step further than the previous one. It focuses your attention while you balance on your toes. Every muscle is pulled up and toned while the mind remains absolutely still. The longer you stand on your toes, the more in control of your body you will be. It is very important to lift the muscle above the kneecaps as you stretch. This will help you to keep your balance.

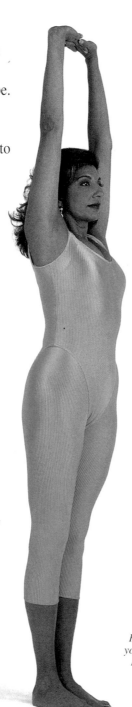

Stand with your feet together and arms stretched above your head. Clasp your fingertips together, keeping your elbows straight.

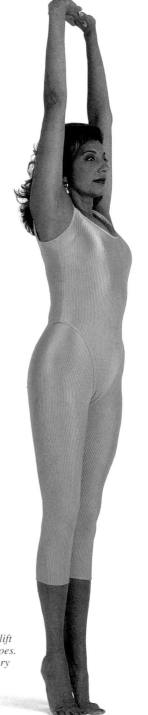

2

Focusing your attention ahead, lift your heels and balance on your toes. Keep reaching upward with every muscle in your body.

Side Stretch

Stretching to the side is an essential movement to maintain mobility and a youthful appearance. The Side Stretch streamlines the waist and trims excess fat from the hips and the thighs. You should stretch from the hips rather than from the waist, keeping your hips square and your feet firmly planted on the floor. It is important not to lean forward. Imagine you are stretching from your toes to your fingertips.

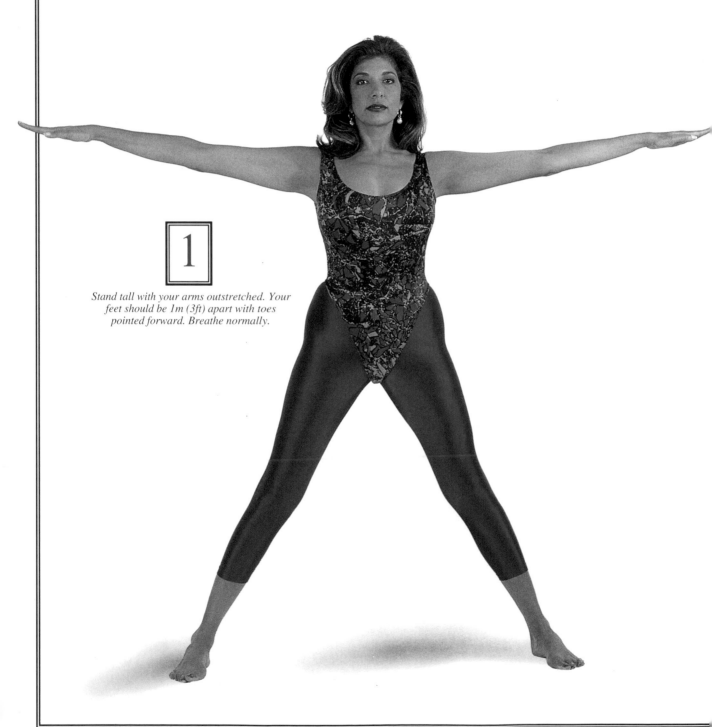

1

Stand tall with your arms outstretched. Your feet should be 1m (3ft) apart with toes pointed forward. Breathe normally.

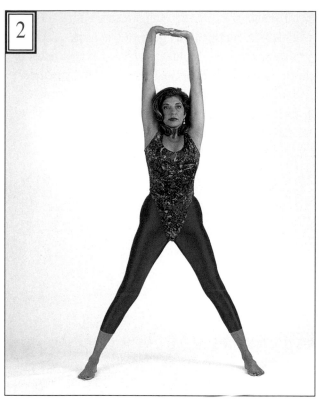

Inhale and bring your arms up over your head. Stretch up as far as you are able with palms face-up and fingers interlaced.

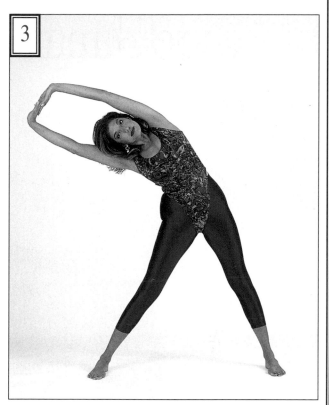

Exhale and stretch to the right. Keep your weight even and push your heels and toes down. Breathe normally and hold for 10 seconds.

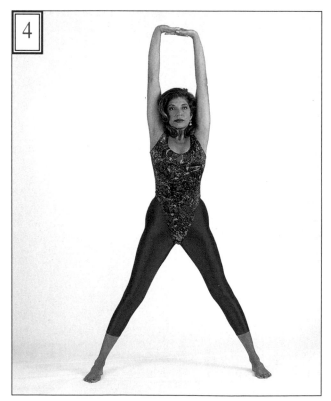

Return to Step 2. Keep stretching from the lower back along the whole spine.

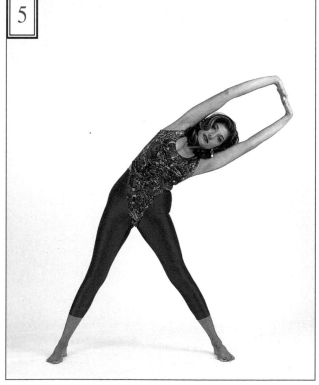

Exhale and stretch over to the left. Breathe normally and hold for 10 seconds. Return to Step 1 and relax.

The Triangle

The Triangle goes a stage further than the Side Stretch and brings more flexibility to the leg muscles and hips. Stretching the spine laterally on both sides increases its elasticity and tones the spinal nerves, helping to relieve backache and neck sprains. The Triangle also develops the chest muscles, tones the abdominal organs and increases stamina. This exercise appears very simple but it is actually more difficult than it looks to get the arm in a straight line with the flat back, as in Step 4.

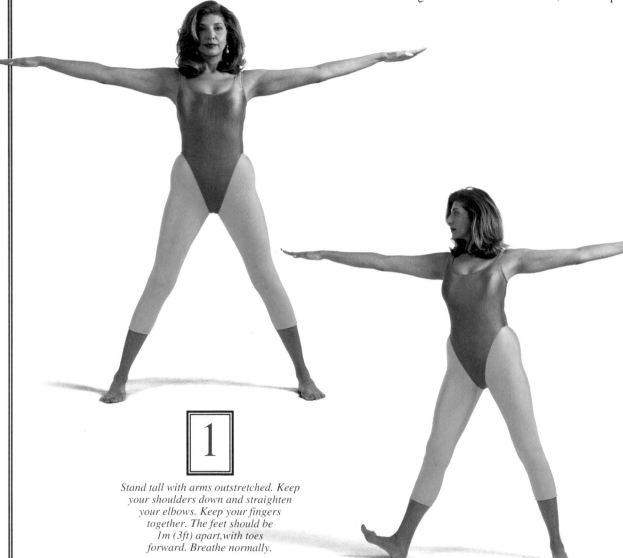

1

Stand tall with arms outstretched. Keep your shoulders down and straighten your elbows. Keep your fingers together. The feet should be 1m (3ft) apart, with toes forward. Breathe normally.

2

Turn your right foot 90° and your left foot slightly inward. The heel of your right foot should align with the left instep.

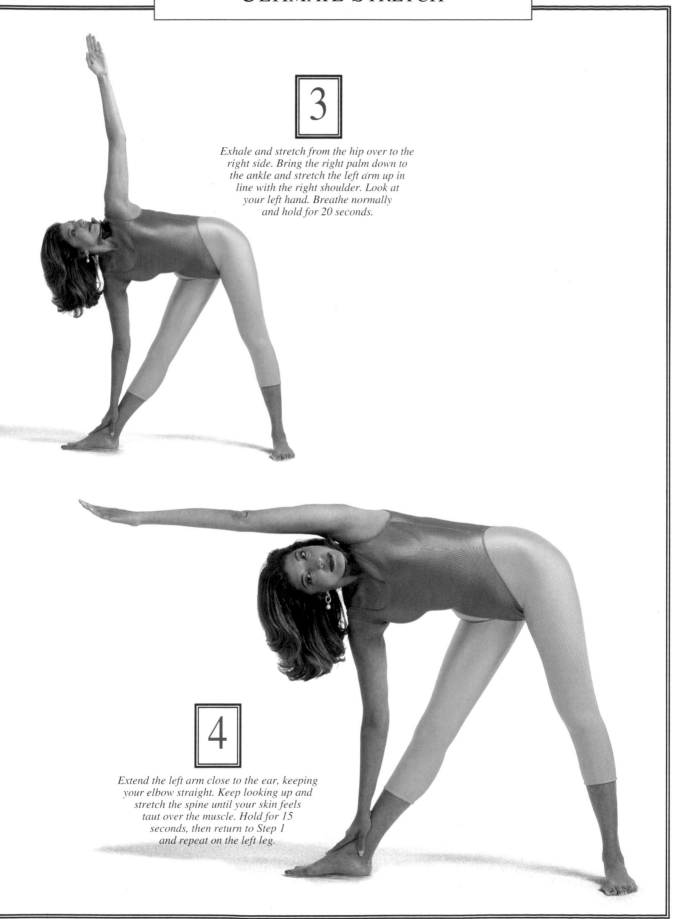

3

Exhale and stretch from the hip over to the right side. Bring the right palm down to the ankle and stretch the left arm up in line with the right shoulder. Look at your left hand. Breathe normally and hold for 20 seconds.

4

Extend the left arm close to the ear, keeping your elbow straight. Keep looking up and stretch the spine until your skin feels taut over the muscle. Hold for 15 seconds, then return to Step 1 and repeat on the left leg.

Head to Knee Side Stretches

These stretches strengthen the legs and improve balance and concentration. While the head is resting on the knee the abdominal organs contract and are toned. The flow of fresh oxygen revitalizes, cleanses and purifies these organs. When performing these exercises, make sure you keep your hips and torso facing directly to the side. You will feel a deep stretch in the back of your knee. If you cannot keep your knee straight, bend it as in Step 5.

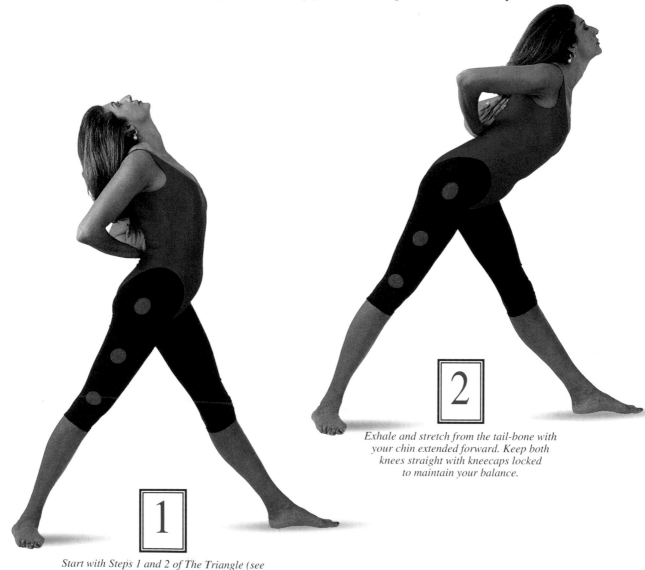

1

Start with Steps 1 and 2 of The Triangle (see page 68), then turn to the side, clasping your hands behind you. Look up, creating an arch in your back, and inhale.

2

Exhale and stretch from the tail-bone with your chin extended forward. Keep both knees straight with kneecaps locked to maintain your balance.

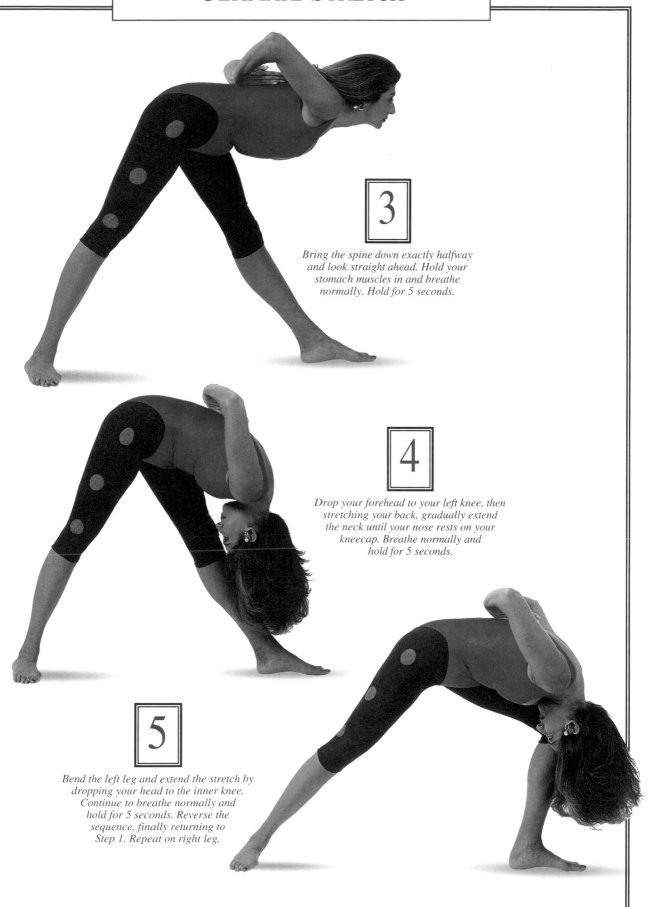

3

Bring the spine down exactly halfway and look straight ahead. Hold your stomach muscles in and breathe normally. Hold for 5 seconds.

4

Drop your forehead to your left knee, then stretching your back, gradually extend the neck until your nose rests on your kneecap. Breathe normally and hold for 5 seconds.

5

Bend the left leg and extend the stretch by dropping your head to the inner knee. Continue to breathe normally and hold for 5 seconds. Reverse the sequence, finally returning to Step 1. Repeat on right leg.

Standing Twist

The Standing Twist is a 'revolving triangle' exercise, which helps to relieve certain back problems, especially lumbago and sciatica. It also strengthens the leg muscles, invigorates the abdominal organs and increases flexibility of the hips. Keep the legs straight and as you bend forward from the lower back slide your hand down your leg to the ankle. Grip the back of your ankle and twist up as much as you can.

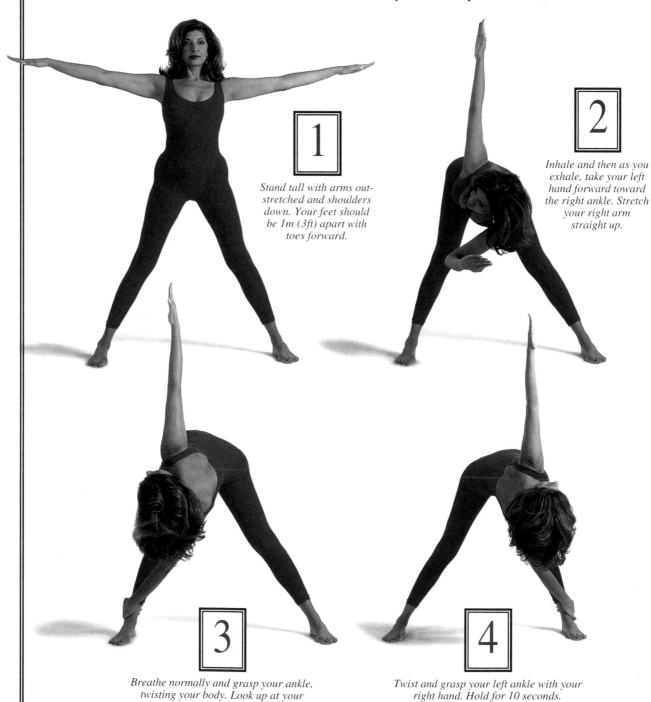

1
Stand tall with arms out-stretched and shoulders down. Your feet should be 1m (3ft) apart with toes forward.

2
Inhale and then as you exhale, take your left hand forward toward the right ankle. Stretch your right arm straight up.

3
Breathe normally and grasp your ankle, twisting your body. Look up at your right thumb. Hold for 10 seconds.

4
Twist and grasp your left ankle with your right hand. Hold for 10 seconds. Return to Step 1 and relax.

The Warrior

The Warrior is a dynamic stretch that creates confidence and poise. It may look simple but staying in exact alignment is not easy. Yogacise teaches discipline of movement and every detail must be be followed for the maximum benefit. During the lunge the knee should be above the foot and no further forward as this can put strain on the knee – you should try to achieve a 90° angle between the thigh and the lower leg.

Stand tall with arms outstretched, shoulders down, elbows straight and fingers together. Your feet should be 1.2m (4ft) apart.

Turn your right foot 90° and your left foot slightly inward. The right heel should be in line with the instep of the left foot. Look beyond your right hand.

Lunge with your right knee until your right thigh is parallel with the floor. Keep your spine upright and your left leg straight with the foot flat on the floor. Hold for 10–15 seconds. Repeat the exercise on the left leg.

Extended Warrior

This intense stretch tones every muscle and tendon in the body. It trims the upper thighs, the hips and the waistline, invigorates the internal organs and soothes the nerves. It is also very beneficial to the endocrine system, consisting of the pituitary, thyroid, pancreas and gonad glands which secrete hormones. Yogic postures help to strengthen the endocrine system and bring the emotions under control.

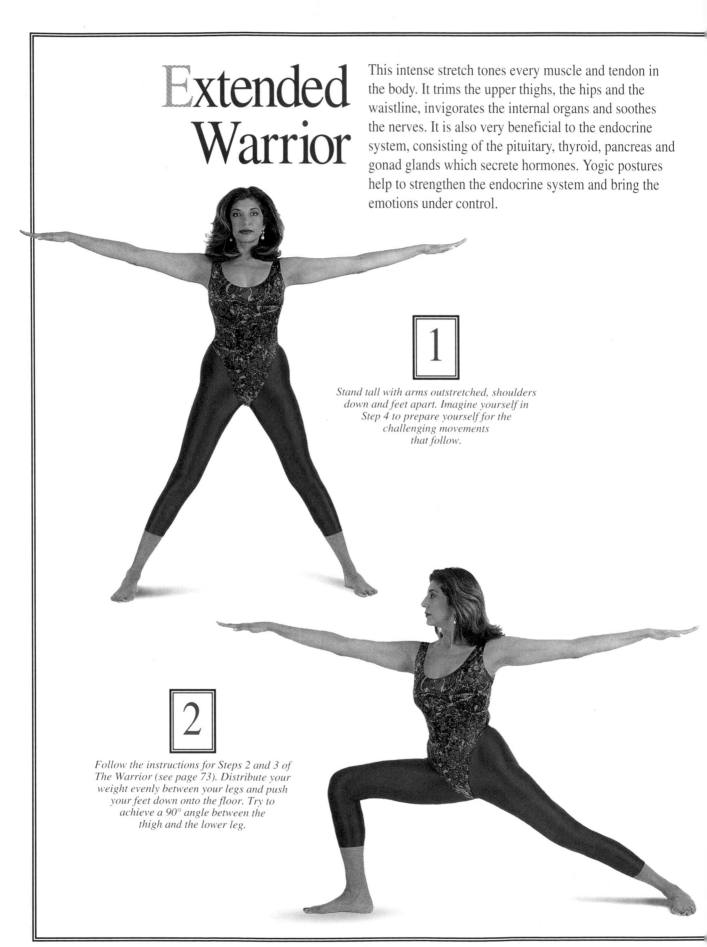

1

Stand tall with arms outstretched, shoulders down and feet apart. Imagine yourself in Step 4 to prepare yourself for the challenging movements that follow.

2

Follow the instructions for Steps 2 and 3 of The Warrior (see page 73). Distribute your weight evenly between your legs and push your feet down onto the floor. Try to achieve a 90° angle between the thigh and the lower leg.

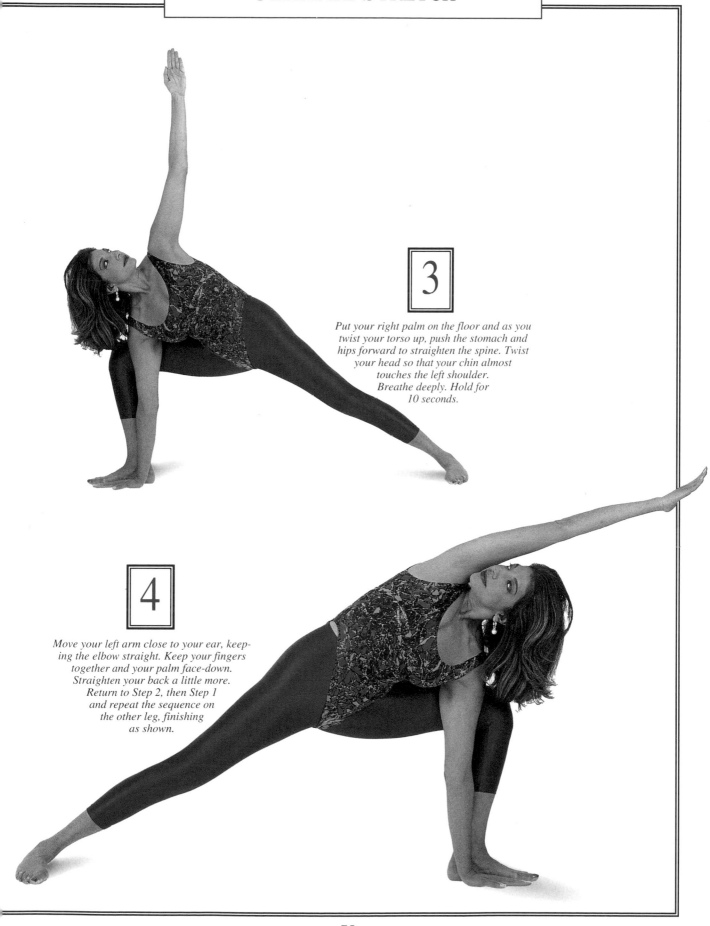

3

Put your right palm on the floor and as you twist your torso up, push the stomach and hips forward to straighten the spine. Twist your head so that your chin almost touches the left shoulder. Breathe deeply. Hold for 10 seconds.

4

Move your left arm close to your ear, keeping the elbow straight. Keep your fingers together and your palm face-down. Straighten your back a little more. Return to Step 2, then Step 1 and repeat the sequence on the other leg, finishing as shown.

Head to Floor Stretch

Stretching forward from the hips has a profound effect on the central nervous system. Flexibility increases in the hamstrings and hips and the spine is invigorated due to increased circulation. It is very important to think of 'lengthening' from the tail-bone rather than from the waist. Always keep the back straight and relax smoothly and gently into the stretch. Never bounce or make any sudden, jerky movements.

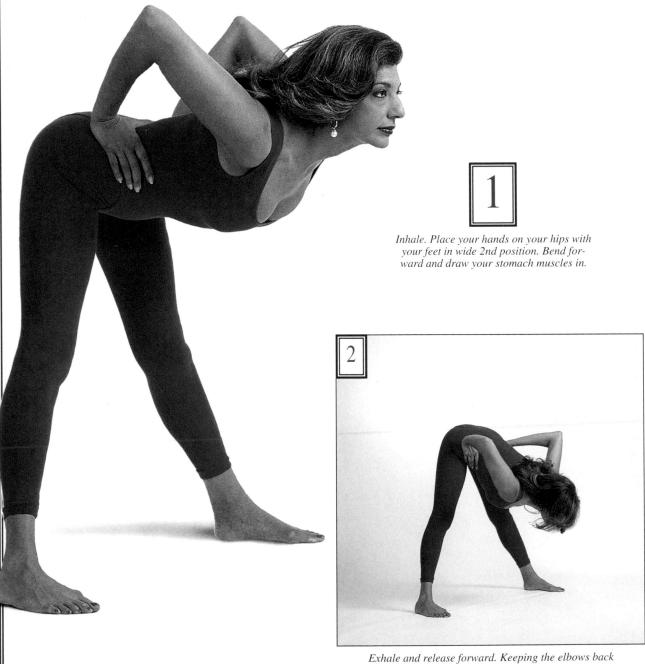

1

Inhale. Place your hands on your hips with your feet in wide 2nd position. Bend forward and draw your stomach muscles in.

2

Exhale and release forward. Keeping the elbows back will help to open up your chest.

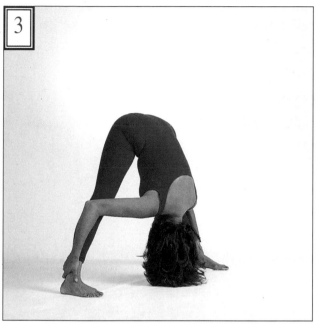

Take hold of your ankles and drop down as far as you find comfortable, bending your elbows as you do so.

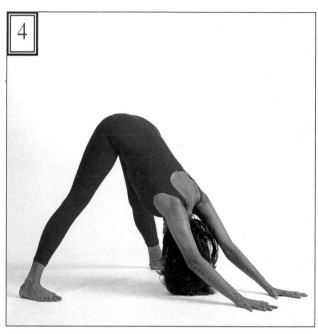

With palms flat on the floor walk your hands as far in front of you as you can, stretching your spine. Hold for 30 seconds.

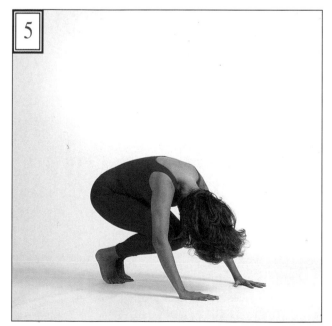

Walk your hands back, exhale and jump your feet together into 1st position with your heels raised.

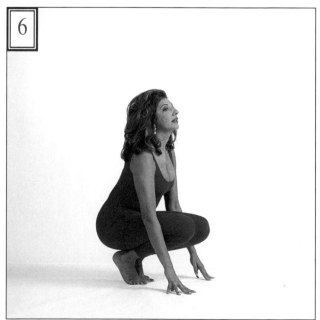

Inhale, straighten your back and balance on your toes. Then stand up, gently uncurling your spine.

Sitting Side Stretch

It is vital to learn how to stretch properly. The normal tendency is to collapse at the waist and curve the spine but you should avoid this as it compresses the front of the body and can strain the ligaments and put pressure on the spinal discs. Instead, you should stretch from the tail-bone and lengthen forward. As you stretch forward you improve circulation to the kidneys and eliminate many harmful toxins from the body. Your internal organs and abdominal muscles are toned. Back problems are relieved as you stimulate the sciatica nerve, and flexibility is increased especially in the hips, hamstrings and spine.

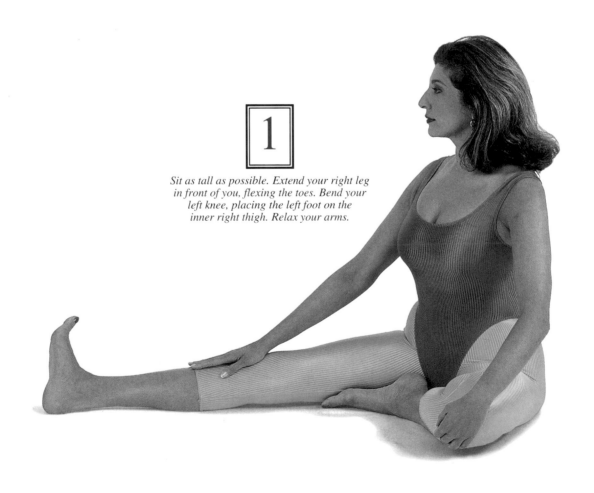

1

Sit as tall as possible. Extend your right leg in front of you, flexing the toes. Bend your left knee, placing the left foot on the inner right thigh. Relax your arms.

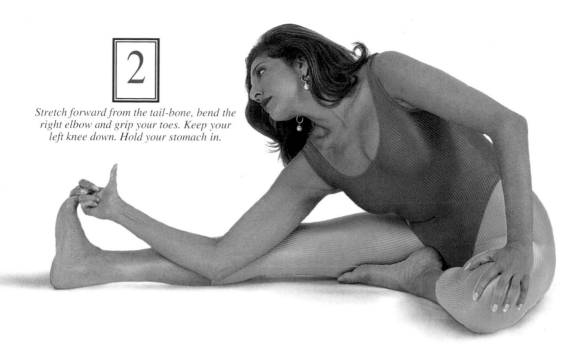

2

Stretch forward from the tail-bone, bend the right elbow and grip your toes. Keep your left knee down. Hold your stomach in.

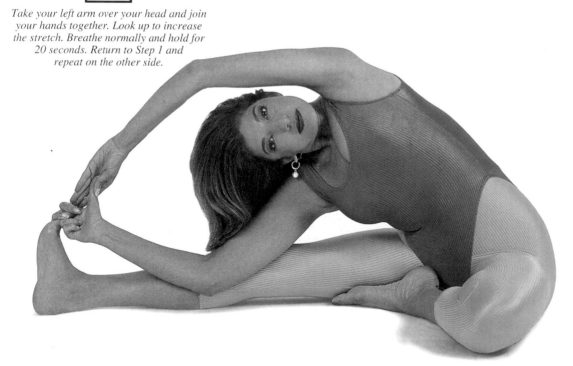

3

Take your left arm over your head and join your hands together. Look up to increase the stretch. Breathe normally and hold for 20 seconds. Return to Step 1 and repeat on the other side.

Hip and Thigh Side Stretch

Many people will find it difficult at first to sit upright in a wide 2nd position because their abdominal and lower back muscles are weak. As you perform this stretch, keep turning the thighs back and pushing the

kneecaps down. You should not see any space under the knees. If you are unable to grasp your big toe in Step 2, instead you should hold the knee with your right hand and stretch your left arm close to your ear.

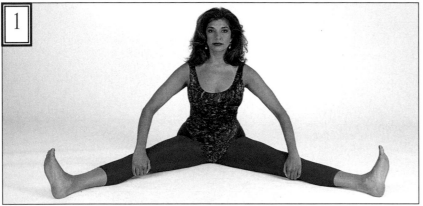

Sit upright and push your tail-bone down on the floor. Bring your legs apart into 2nd position. Breathe normally, then inhale and slowly exhale.

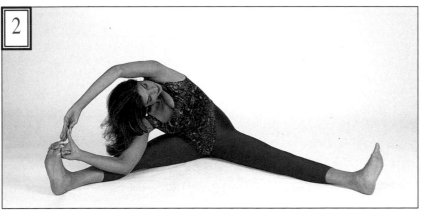

Exhale and bending to the right, bring your left arm over. Clasp your fingers, and if possible, your big toe. Breathe deeply for 10 seconds.

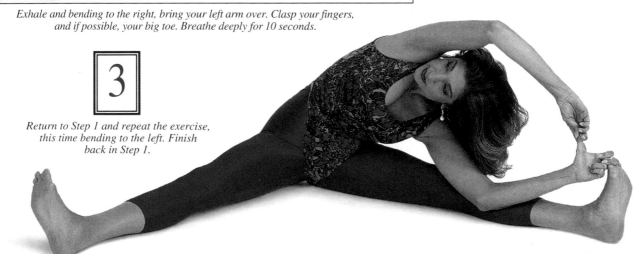

Return to Step 1 and repeat the exercise, this time bending to the left. Finish back in Step 1.

Spine Stretch

Only with practice and perseverance will your hips and thighs become supple enough to enable you to do this exercise and achieve the aim of this exercise – to bring your head forward to the floor. Do not make any jerking movements. Breathe deeply and relax in Step 3 to increase flexibility.

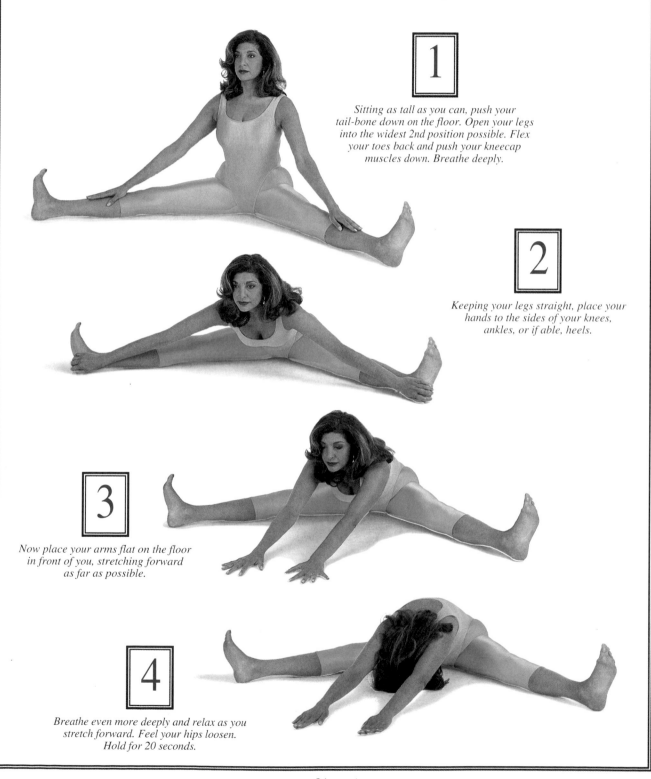

1

Sitting as tall as you can, push your tail-bone down on the floor. Open your legs into the widest 2nd position possible. Flex your toes back and push your kneecap muscles down. Breathe deeply.

2

Keeping your legs straight, place your hands to the sides of your knees, ankles, or if able, heels.

3

Now place your arms flat on the floor in front of you, stretching forward as far as possible.

4

Breathe even more deeply and relax as you stretch forward. Feel your hips loosen. Hold for 20 seconds.

Hip Opener

This stretch is specifically designed to work on the hip joints. Leaning forward in this position acts as a natural weight to gently open up the hips and thighs. As you perform the Hip Opener, you should breathe deeply from the diaphragm to loosen and relax the muscles.

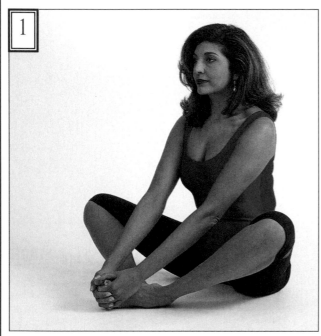

Bring the soles of your feet together and hold onto your toes. Breathe normally.

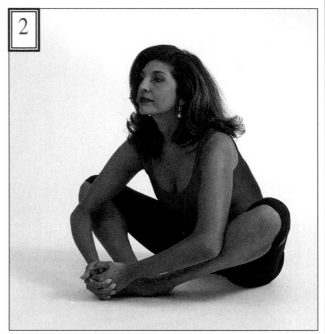

Lean forward, keeping your back flat. Lift your chin forward. When you reach your maximum stretch, relax down.

Drop your forehead slowly down toward your feet. Try to push your knees open without forcing them. Hold and breathe deeply for 10 seconds.

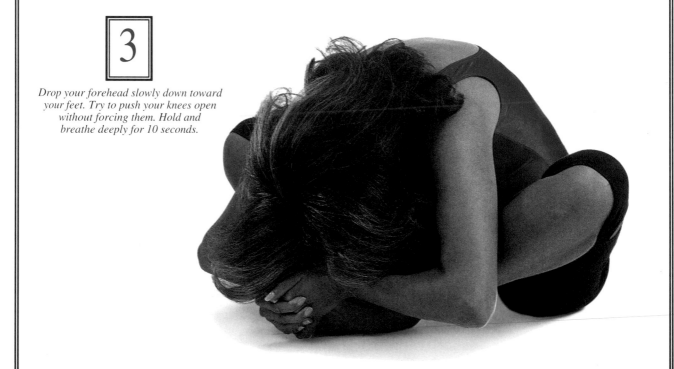

Life Force

This breathing technique centers the body and keeps the mind still. It produces an even flow of energy that helps to relax tight muscles. When you are practising this technique, concentrate on how the energy is flowing throughout your body after the stretching exercises. Adopt a lotus or half-lotus position, or if you find this uncomfortable, try sitting cross-legged or in a chair.

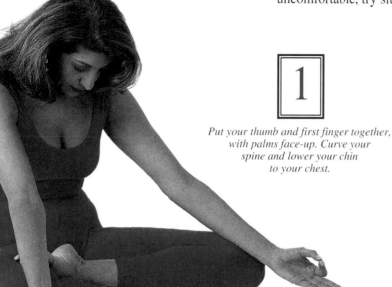

1

Put your thumb and first finger together, with palms face-up. Curve your spine and lower your chin to your chest.

2

Visualize the energy situated at the base of your spine. Slowly inhale and lift your spine in perfect posture. Breathe normally. Straighten your arms and feel the energy moving up your spine through the top of your head and into your fingertips. Remain in this position for 5 minutes or more.

Classical

This chapter is based on the best-known *Hatha* Yoga *asanas* that harmonize the mind and body. The following exercises are designed specifically to build stamina, increase flexibility and suppleness and help focus the mind to improve concentration. You will notice that many of the poses involve balance. Balance comes from a focused mind and the very act of holding a pose for a length of time will force the mind and body to harmonize naturally. The result is a wonderful sense of stillness and calm.

Classical exercises are very challenging and dynamic. You may find them difficult at first but with regular practice you will soon make progress. Always remember to breathe deeply through the nose from the diaphragm. Each *asana* works on specific organs in the body and it is important to breathe correctly so that fresh oxygen is sent to replenish the cells in those organs.

As you experience the joys of mastering these *asanas*, your life will be transformed by a new outlook, better health and a more positive attitude.

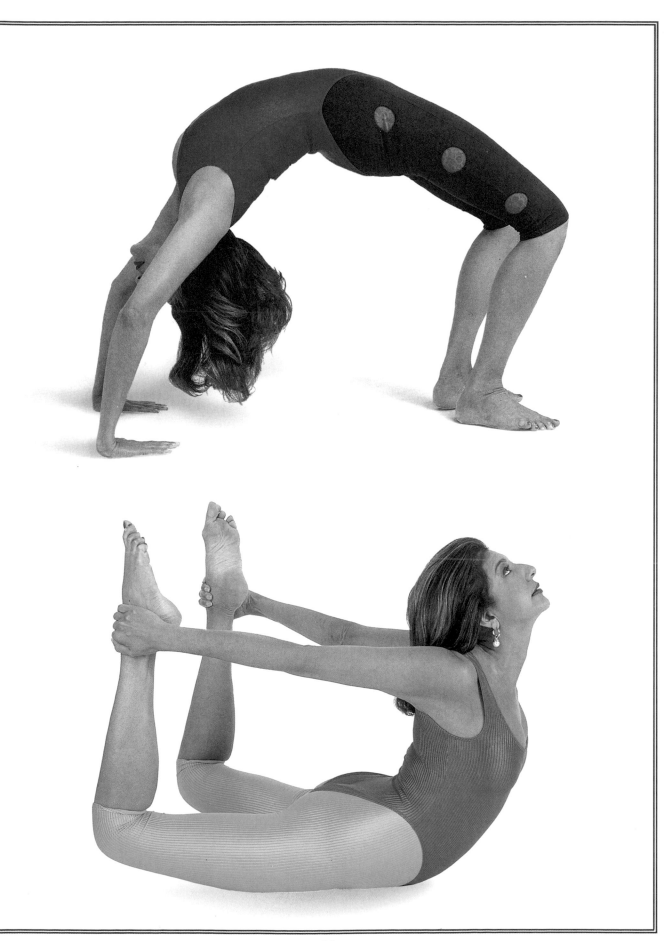

The Eagle

The Eagle requires concentration and flexibility. It strengthens the calf muscles and eliminates surplus fat around the thighs. As you practise, focus on one point ahead of you and try to remain still. This is a 'grounding' exercise, so try to sink deeper and deeper into the standing knee. Breathe normally while holding for as long as possible then repeat on the other leg.

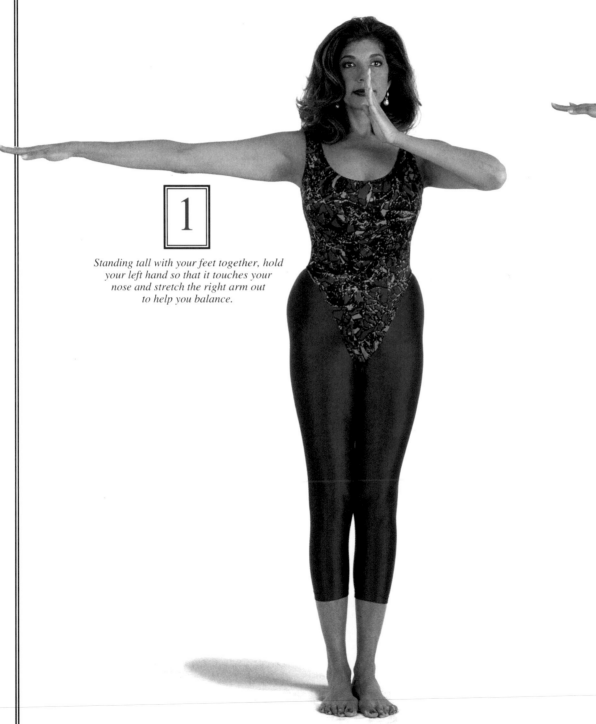

1

Standing tall with your feet together, hold your left hand so that it touches your nose and stretch the right arm out to help you balance.

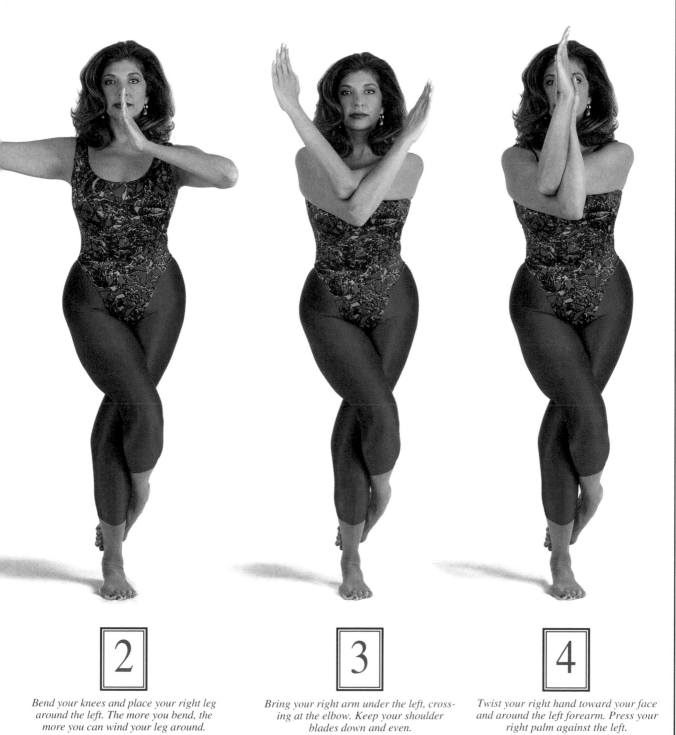

<table>
<tr>
<td style="text-align:center">2</td>
<td style="text-align:center">3</td>
<td style="text-align:center">4</td>
</tr>
</table>

Bend your knees and place your right leg around the left. The more you bend, the more you can wind your leg around.

Bring your right arm under the left, crossing at the elbow. Keep your shoulder blades down and even.

Twist your right hand toward your face and around the left forearm. Press your right palm against the left.

The Standing Bow

The Standing Bow is one of the most difficult classical positions because it combines balance, flexibility, stamina and strength. The pose helps you to develop concentration and determination. It also transfers the circulation from one side of the body to the other. The energy moves full circle, so that your body is revitalized and rejuvenated. In addition, the rib cage and lungs expand while the lower back increases in strength and flexibility. This exercise will also improve your muscle tone, increase your circulation and help reduce cellulite.

The challenge is to hold the position for as long as you can, so whenever

1

Standing tall, focus ahead. Balance on the left leg. Raise your right leg behind you, holding the foot on the inside.

2

Lift your left arm to help you balance. Keep your elbows straight, fingertips pointed upward, and hips square. Inhale.

3

Exhale. Kick your leg upward and back with all your strength. Hold the middle of the foot tightly.

you practice, set yourself a goal and try to increase the time you hold the final pose. You will find that the body, when in perfect alignment, will balance for a considerable period.

The Standing Bow looks static but is actually a total stretch that continues to move while in the position. Think of your body as an elastic band, pulling from one side to another. The way to increase the total stretch is to point your toes and stretch your arm forward, creating a 90° angle between your arm, body and leg.

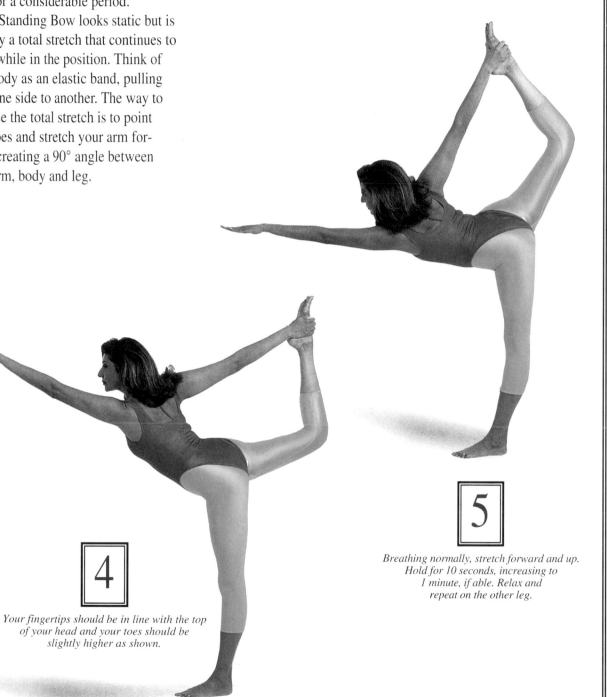

4

Your fingertips should be in line with the top of your head and your toes should be slightly higher as shown.

5

Breathing normally, stretch forward and up. Hold for 10 seconds, increasing to 1 minute, if able. Relax and repeat on the other leg.

Head to Knee

Head to Knee is one of the most difficult standing postures and is, not surprisingly, a tremendous challenge. In common with the Standing Bow it develops concentration, balance, flexibility and stamina. Do not be discouraged if you cannot progress beyond Step 1 for some time. The most important point to remember is to keep the leg that you are standing on straight.

Stand tall with feet together. Inhale and lift the right knee up to the chest. Breathe normally and hold for 10 seconds.

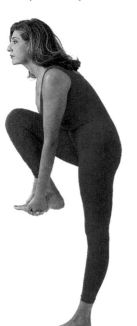

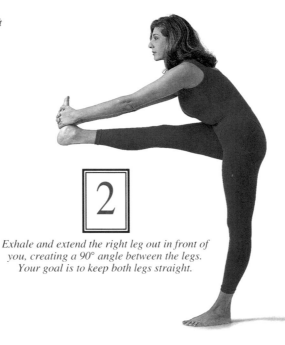

Exhale and extend the right leg out in front of you, creating a 90° angle between the legs. Your goal is to keep both legs straight.

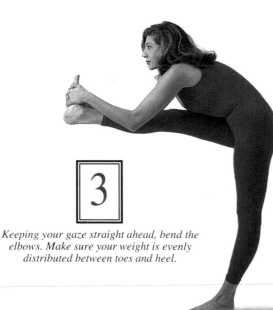

Keeping your gaze straight ahead, bend the elbows. Make sure your weight is evenly distributed between toes and heel.

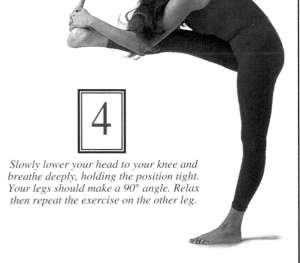

Slowly lower your head to your knee and breathe deeply, holding the position tight. Your legs should make a 90° angle. Relax then repeat the exercise on the other leg.

Toe Balance

This posture teaches concentration and patience. When you lift the spine upright and the body grows into perfect alignment you feel weightless. Your mind and body harmonize and you experience a sense of elation. The Toe Balance also helps to alleviate arthritis of the knees and ankles. Breathe normally throughout the exercise.

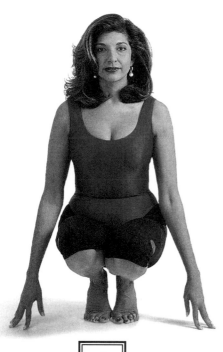

1

Begin by centering yourself and balancing on your toes. Place your fingertips on the floor to help you balance.

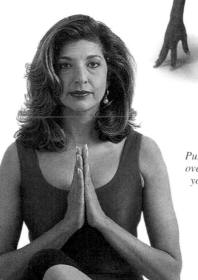

2

Push your left leg forward, placing the knee over your right leg. Lift your spine as far as you can. Balance on the ball of your foot.

3

When you feel balanced, bring your palms together. Hold for 10 seconds and then repeat the exercise on the other leg.

Shoulder Stand

The Shoulder Stand provides the thyroid with a rich supply of blood. The thyroid, situated in the neck, is the most important gland in the endocrine system – it controls the metabolism that stabilizes weight gain or loss and also corrects hormonal imbalance.

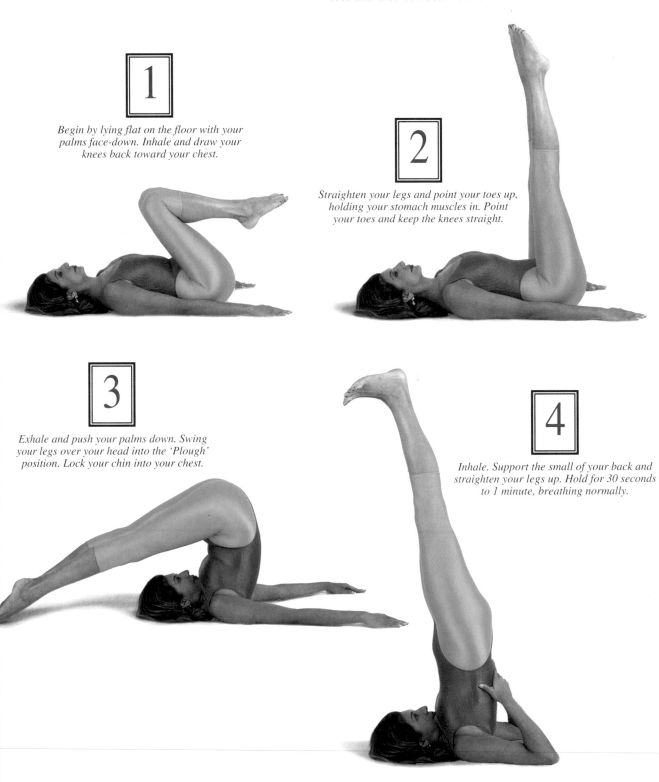

1

Begin by lying flat on the floor with your palms face-down. Inhale and draw your knees back toward your chest.

2

Straighten your legs and point your toes up, holding your stomach muscles in. Point your toes and keep the knees straight.

3

Exhale and push your palms down. Swing your legs over your head into the 'Plough' position. Lock your chin into your chest.

4

Inhale. Support the small of your back and straighten your legs up. Hold for 30 seconds to 1 minute, breathing normally.

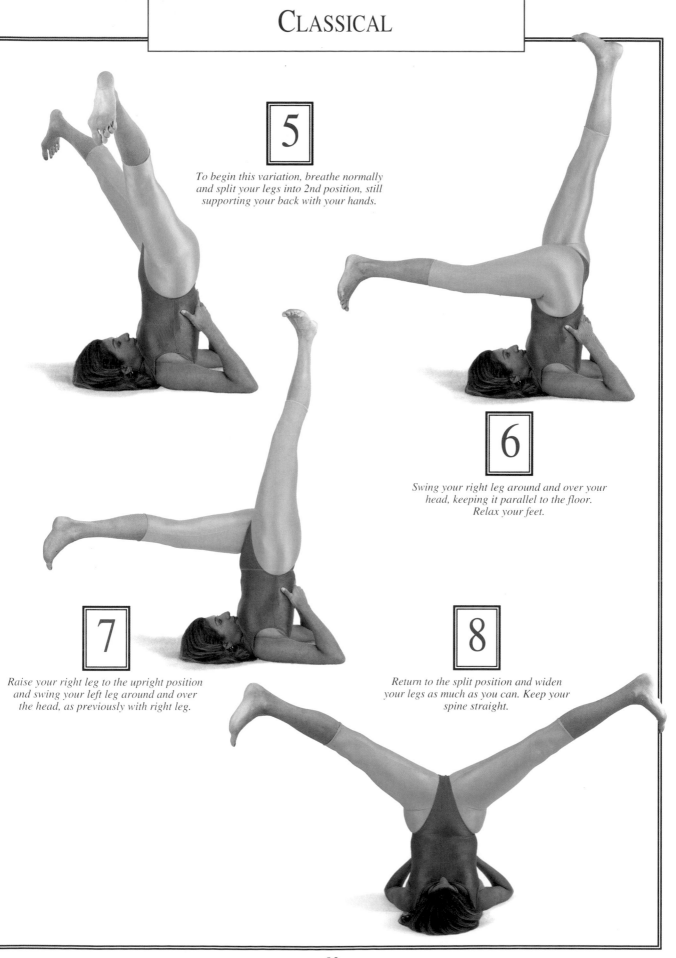

5

To begin this variation, breathe normally and split your legs into 2nd position, still supporting your back with your hands.

6

Swing your right leg around and over your head, keeping it parallel to the floor. Relax your feet.

7

Raise your right leg to the upright position and swing your left leg around and over the head, as previously with right leg.

8

Return to the split position and widen your legs as much as you can. Keep your spine straight.

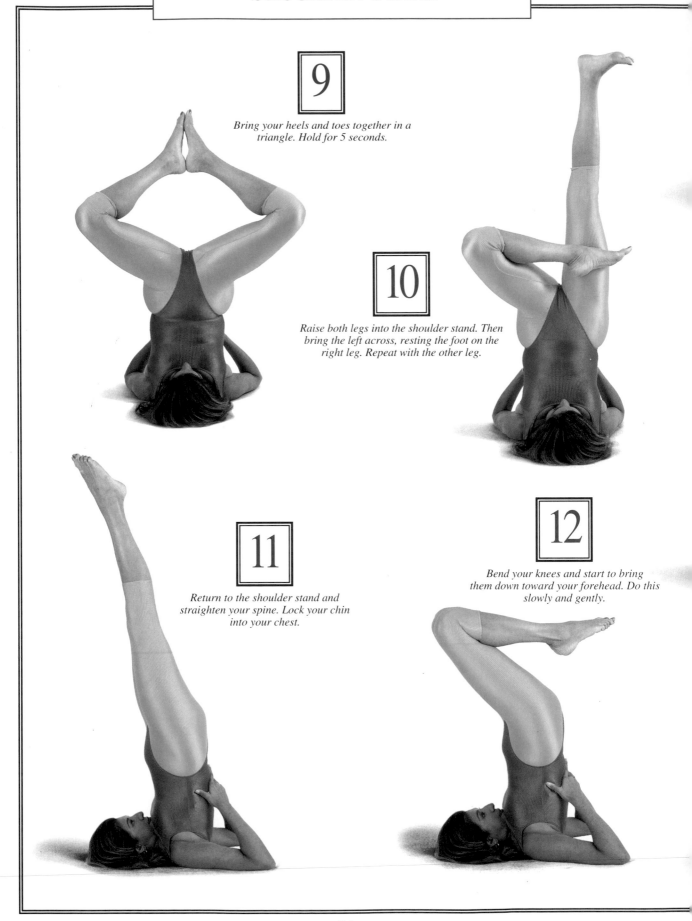

9

Bring your heels and toes together in a triangle. Hold for 5 seconds.

10

Raise both legs into the shoulder stand. Then bring the left across, resting the foot on the right leg. Repeat with the other leg.

11

Return to the shoulder stand and straighten your spine. Lock your chin into your chest.

12

Bend your knees and start to bring them down toward your forehead. Do this slowly and gently.

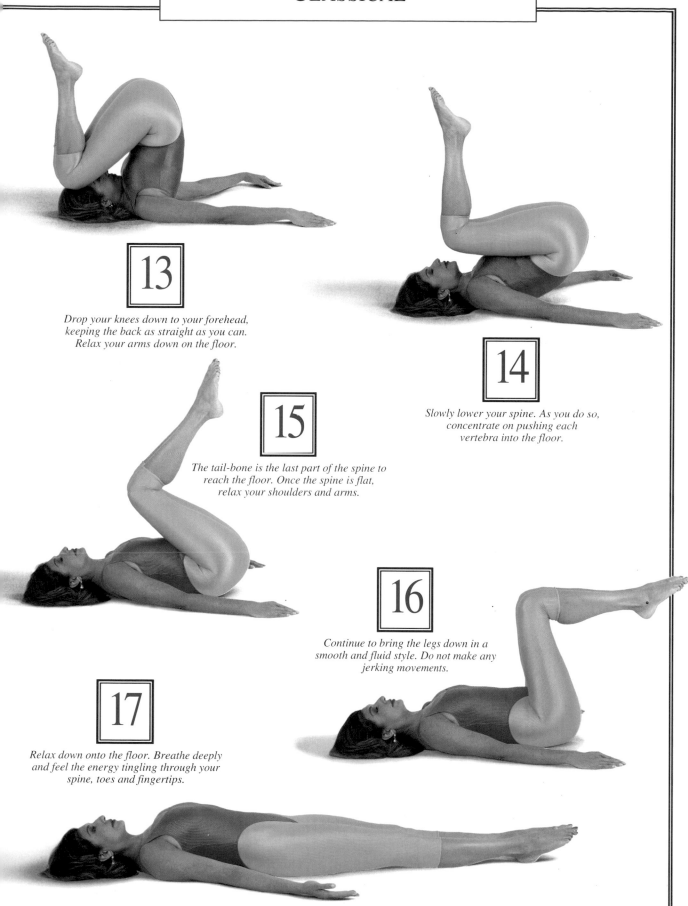

13

Drop your knees down to your forehead, keeping the back as straight as you can. Relax your arms down on the floor.

14

Slowly lower your spine. As you do so, concentrate on pushing each vertebra into the floor.

15

The tail-bone is the last part of the spine to reach the floor. Once the spine is flat, relax your shoulders and arms.

16

Continue to bring the legs down in a smooth and fluid style. Do not make any jerking movements.

17

Relax down onto the floor. Breathe deeply and feel the energy tingling through your spine, toes and fingertips.

The Fish

The Fish should always follow the Shoulder Stand to counteract the effect of the inverted spine. The chest expands and breathing becomes deeper, the thyroid benefits due to the neck stretching, and the leg and abdominal muscles are toned. The Fish also improves circulation to the face and helps to prevent facial wrinkles and sagging muscles in the neck and throat.

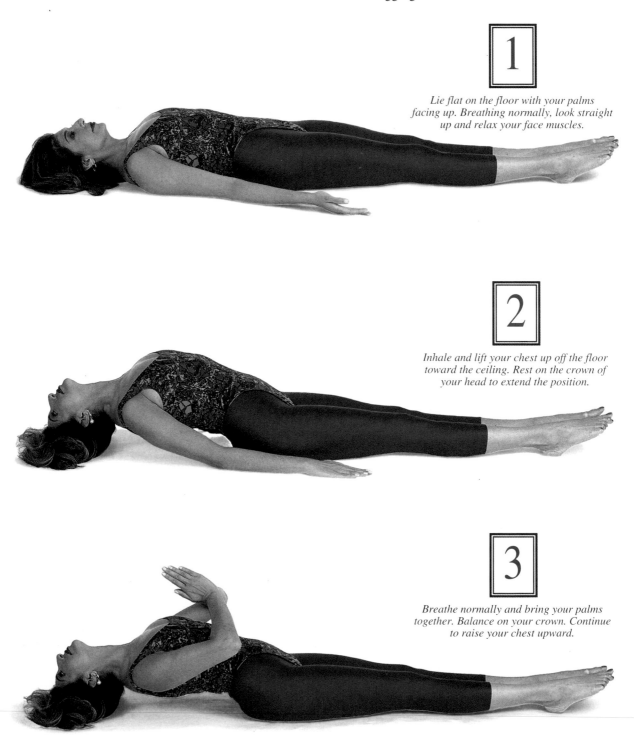

1

Lie flat on the floor with your palms facing up. Breathing normally, look straight up and relax your face muscles.

2

Inhale and lift your chest up off the floor toward the ceiling. Rest on the crown of your head to extend the position.

3

Breathe normally and bring your palms together. Balance on your crown. Continue to raise your chest upward.

4

*Concentrating on your stomach muscles,
inhale and slowly lift your right leg. Hold
for 10 seconds, breathing normally.*

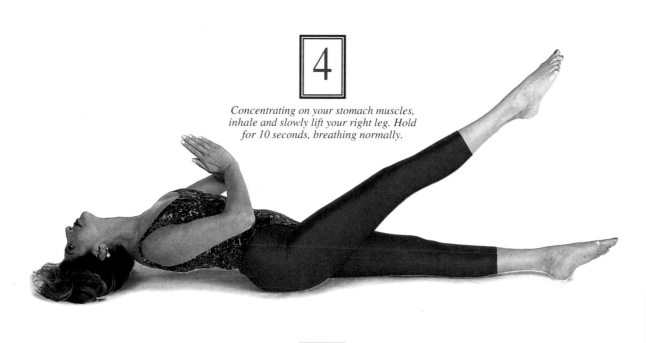

5

*Exhale and slowly lower the right leg.
Inhale and raise the left leg, hold for 10 seconds, then exhale and slowly lower it.*

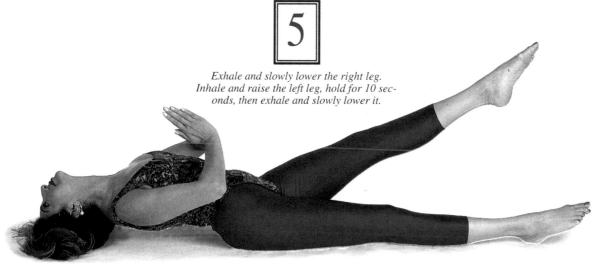

6

*Breathe normally and release your neck and
shoulders. Relax down onto the floor,
breathing deeply.*

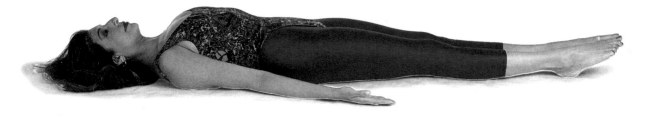

The Wheel

The Wheel is an intense spinal stretch that releases energy in the body's cells, glands and organs. The muscles of the legs, hips, shoulders and arms, along with the spine and its ligaments, receive a complete bend and stretch. This opens the chest, increasing lung capacity. It also helps to alleviate backache.

1

Breathing normally, lie flat with knees bent and feet as close as possible to your backside. Keep your feet in line with your hips.

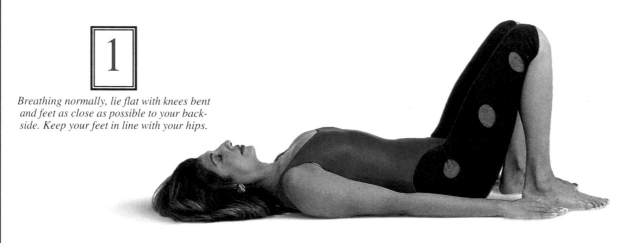

2

Inhale and raise your hips as high as you can. Holding your ankles will increase the stretch. Breathing normally, hold for 10 seconds.

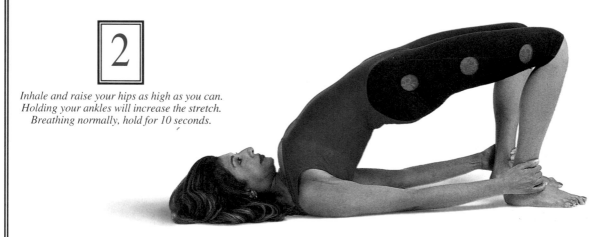

3

Breathing deeply, place your hands beside your head with palms facing down and fingertips facing in toward your ears.

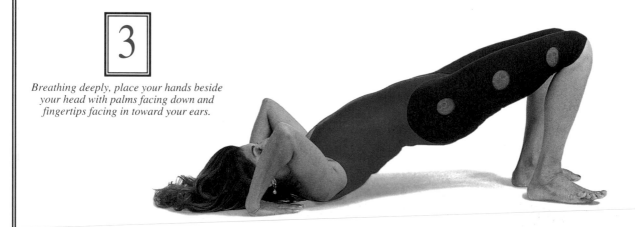

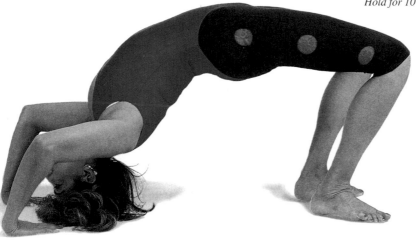

4

Inhale, raising your hips and chest. Lift your head and rest your crown on the floor. Lift the shoulders and lower back and exhale. Hold for 10 seconds, breathing normally.

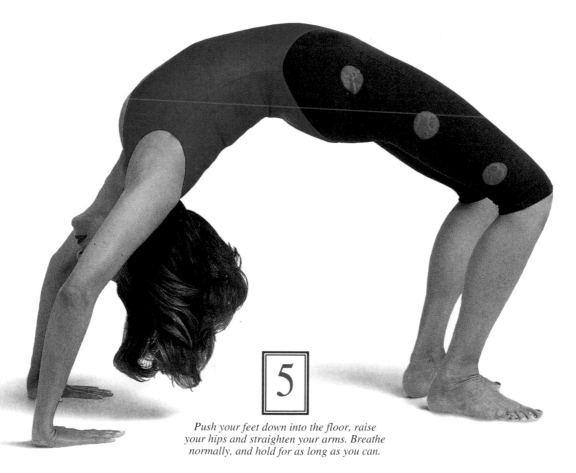

5

Push your feet down into the floor, raise your hips and straighten your arms. Breathe normally, and hold for as long as you can.

The Cobra

The Cobra strengthens the muscles of the lower back, alleviating back pain and enabling you to lift your spine in perfect posture. It also helps to relieve the symptoms of lumbago, rheumatism and arthritis of the spine and regulates the menstrual cycle. Practising The Cobra helps to expand the chest, strengthens the wrists and neck and tones the thyroid and adrenal glands.

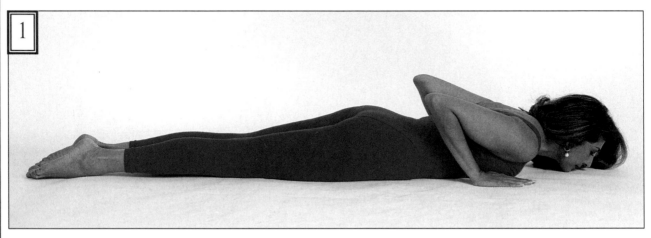

Lying flat with your chin resting on the floor, bring your arms close to the body with your hands under your shoulders.

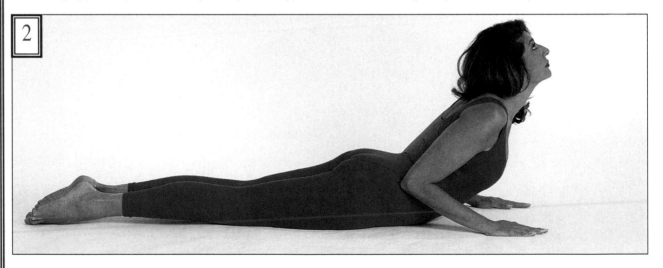

Inhale and push your palms down. Raise your chest off the floor and look upward. Hold for 10 seconds breathing normally.

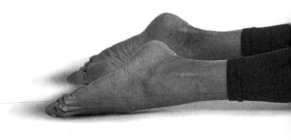

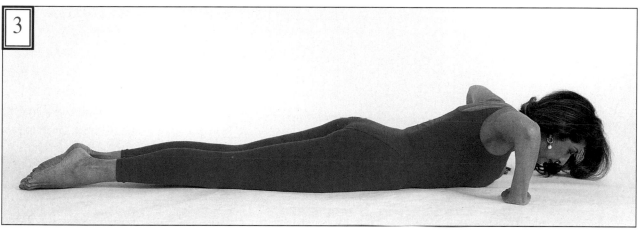

Return to Step 1. Then move your hands so that your fingertips point inward toward your shoulders and your elbows point out.

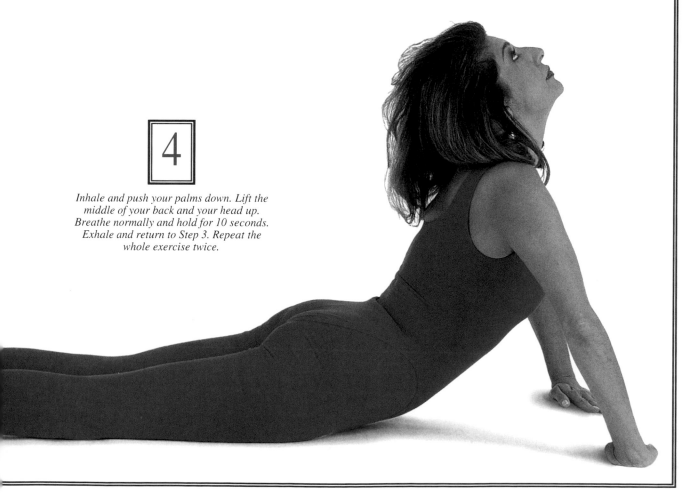

4

Inhale and push your palms down. Lift the middle of your back and your head up. Breathe normally and hold for 10 seconds. Exhale and return to Step 3. Repeat the whole exercise twice.

The Bow

The Bow is a back bend that not only tones every muscle in the body but opens the chest and expands the lungs. This helps achieve a positive outlook and a dynamic quality to life. It awakens the spine without putting strain on the lower back. The upper back and hips stretch in one continuous curve. Increased suppleness releases energy that rejuvenates and revitalizes every cell, helping to keep the body youthful.

Most people do not have an opportunity to bend backward in their daily life. So if you find this exercise difficult, begin by simply lifting your head and feet off the floor. Your goal as you get better at the exercise is to keep the head and knee in a direct line with each other. As you reach up it is important to think of lengthening forward from the upper back, while at the same time kicking the legs upward.

1

Lie flat with your chin resting on the floor.
Bend your knees behind you and hold
onto your ankles.

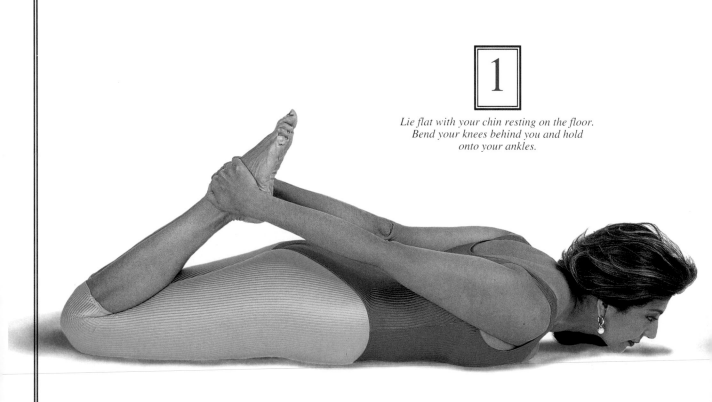

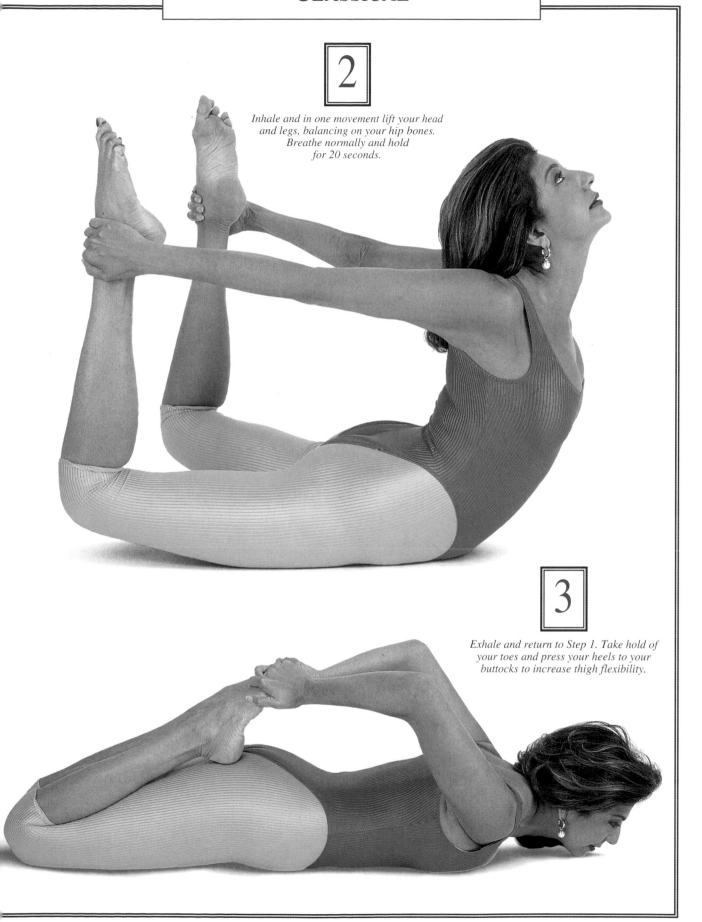

2

Inhale and in one movement lift your head and legs, balancing on your hip bones. Breathe normally and hold for 20 seconds.

3

Exhale and return to Step 1. Take hold of your toes and press your heels to your buttocks to increase thigh flexibility.

The Cat Stretch

After The Bow or other back bend it is important to stretch the spine to release any tension or blockages. When you perform intense back stretches try to make the movement as continuous as possible, otherwise it may result in tightness in some parts of the vertebrae.

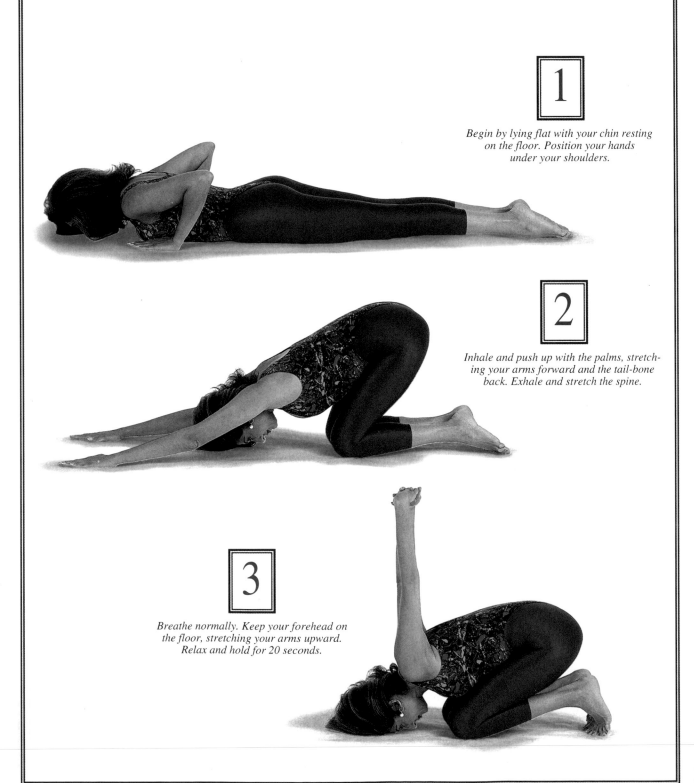

1

Begin by lying flat with your chin resting on the floor. Position your hands under your shoulders.

2

Inhale and push up with the palms, stretching your arms forward and the tail-bone back. Exhale and stretch the spine.

3

Breathe normally. Keep your forehead on the floor, stretching your arms upward. Relax and hold for 20 seconds.

Alternative Nostril Breathing

This is a classical *pranayama* exercise that balances the masculine energy of the right side and the feminine energy of the left. By breathing separately through each nostril you become aware of your breathing and are able to focus your mind. Once you have completed the sequence, repeat Steps 3 and 4 for 10 seconds each.

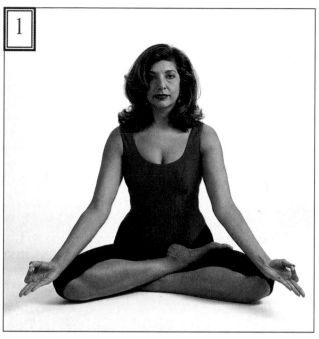

1

Sit tall in a half-lotus or cross-legged position and focus ahead. Join the thumb and first finger. Breathe deeply for 8 seconds.

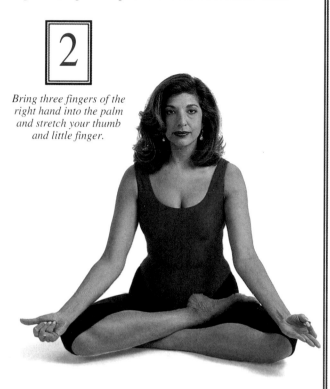

2

Bring three fingers of the right hand into the palm and stretch your thumb and little finger.

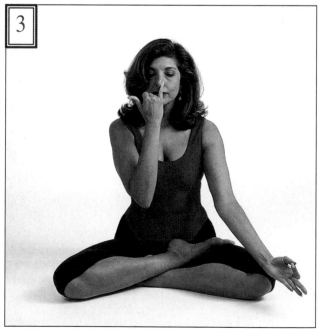

3

Now block the left nostril with the little finger of the right hand and breathe only through the right nostril for 10 seconds.

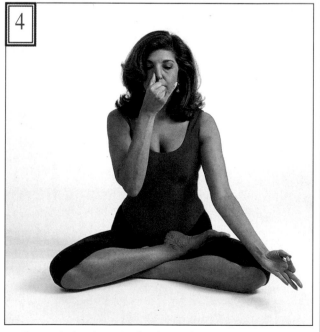

4

Change the hand position by closing the right nostril with the thumb and breathe though the left nostril for 10 seconds.

De-Stress

Everyone experiences stress in varying degrees in everyday life. Situations constantly arise that throw you off balance. Coping with personal relationships, children, a demanding job, or any kind of change is difficult, but there are ways to combat the adverse effects of stress.

There are certain areas of the body where stress is heightened. The neck, shoulders, upper and lower back, abdomen, legs and feet are particularly vulnerable. For example, standing or sitting for a long time causes strain in ankles, swollen feet, frustration, anger and emotional upsets cause stomach pains, indigestion, and ulcers, and tension in the neck and shoulders blocks the circulation to the brain, causing headaches. This chapter teaches the art of relaxation by providing specific poses to tense and release each muscle group. The technique works upward through the body from the toes to the head. When combined with correct breathing, these exercises reduce stress within the physical body and teach you how to draw energies into yourself to create a sense of peace and develop deep powers of concentration.

Yogacise provides the perfect solution because it teaches you how to restore balance and harmony to your life.

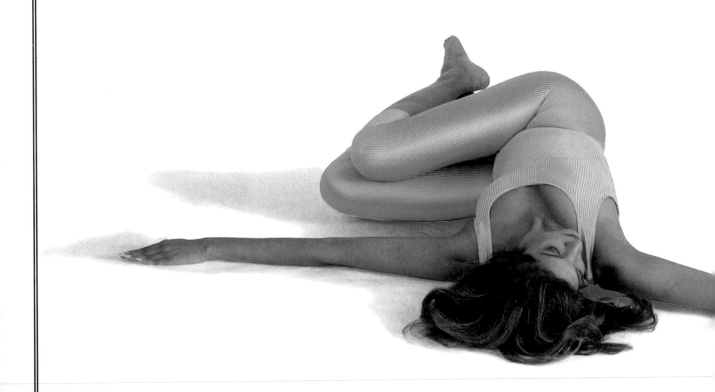

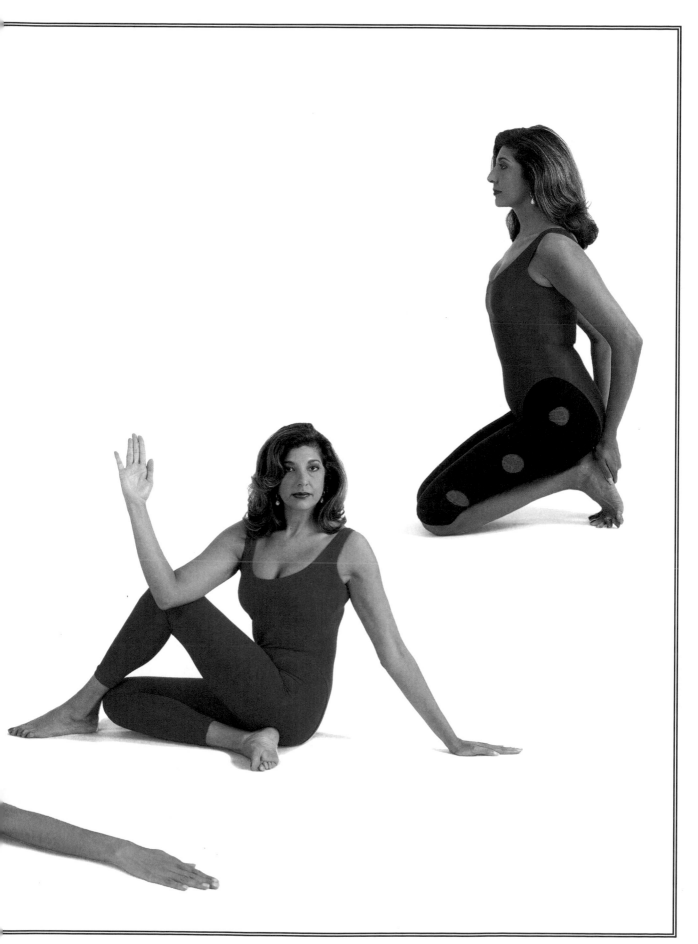

Shoulder Release

Many people experience an ache in the neck and shoulders when they are tense and anxious. This exercise will help you to release tension in that muscle group. Make sure that you start slowly and gradually in order not to sprain already tight muscles. You shouldbe careful to keep your spine straight to isolate the neck and shoulders.

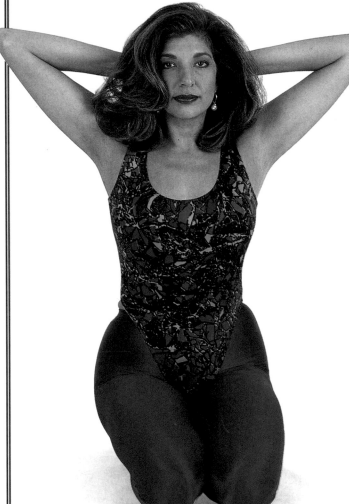

1

Kneeling on the floor and resting on your heels, lift your spine up as tall as you can. Clasp the fingertips together behind your head and raise your elbows so they are even with each other and the forearms are parallel to the floor. Inhale slowly.

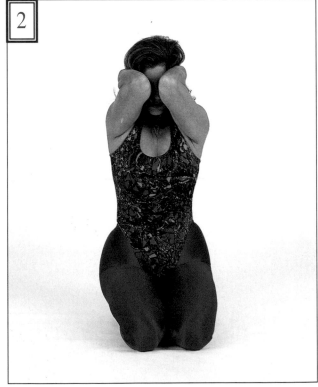

2

Exhale and bring the elbows toward each other. Keep the spine tall and only move your arms.

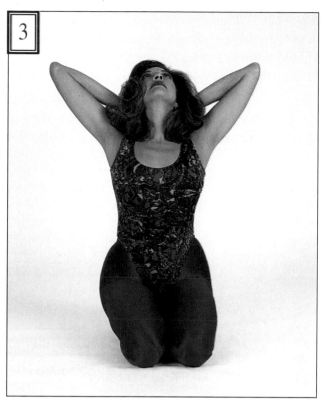

Inhale and look up to the ceiling. Open the elbows and do not curve the spine.

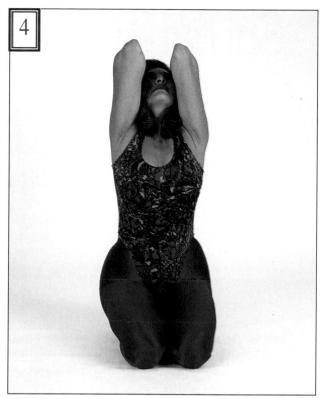

Exhale and bring the elbows together pointing them upward to the ceiling.

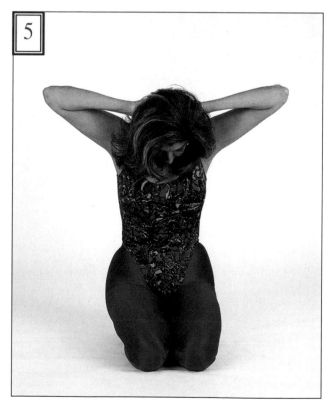

Inhale and look down toward the thighs. Open your elbows and make sure they stay up and back. Keep your shoulders down.

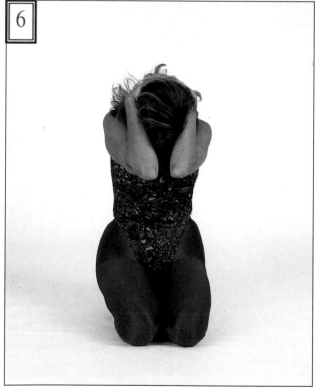

Exhale and bring the elbows together. Do not drop your shoulders or curve the spine. Repeat the whole exercise 4 times.

Spinal Twist 1

Stress causes the body to produce toxins in the internal organs. Spinal twists help to eliminate toxins in the kidneys, liver, stomach and spleen. Spinal twists also increase the mobility of the spine and help to alleviate back pain by relieving stiffness in the feet and the upper and lower back.

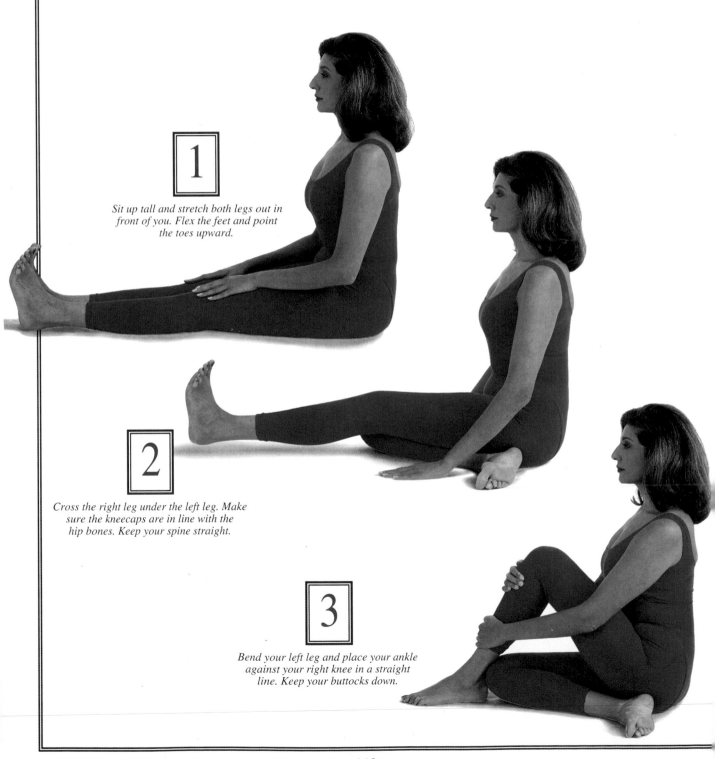

1

Sit up tall and stretch both legs out in front of you. Flex the feet and point the toes upward.

2

Cross the right leg under the left leg. Make sure the kneecaps are in line with the hip bones. Keep your spine straight.

3

Bend your left leg and place your ankle against your right knee in a straight line. Keep your buttocks down.

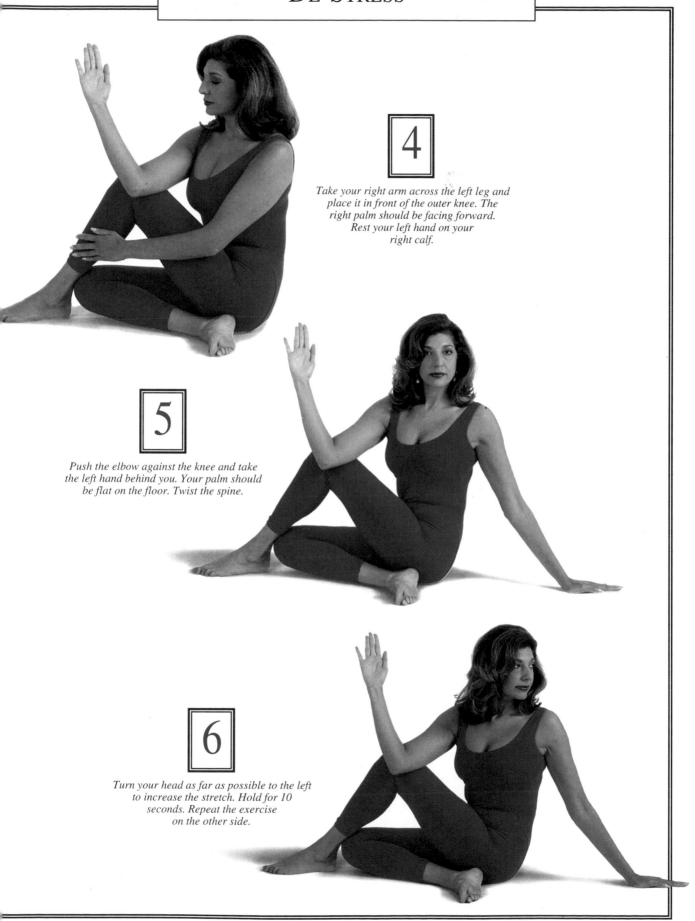

4

Take your right arm across the left leg and
place it in front of the outer knee. The
right palm should be facing forward.
Rest your left hand on your
right calf.

5

Push the elbow against the knee and take
the left hand behind you. Your palm should
be flat on the floor. Twist the spine.

6

Turn your head as far as possible to the left
to increase the stretch. Hold for 10
seconds. Repeat the exercise
on the other side.

Spinal Twist 2

When the body is given a side twist the spine becomes more supple. The muscles of the back are stimulated and the abdominal wall is toned. When the leg and foot are placed on the inner thigh in a half-lotus position, tremendous pressure is placed on the liver and stomach, and some pressure is also placed on the kidneys and intestines. This means that all of the abdominal organs are massaged and circulation is increased, helping to eliminate poisons that are produced in the digestive process. If you find the half-lotus in Step 1 too difficult, place your foot on the inner thigh instead. If you cannot reach the back of the foot in Step 5, then place your hands on your knee or ankle. Breathe nor-mally throughout the sequence and hold each position for 5 seconds.

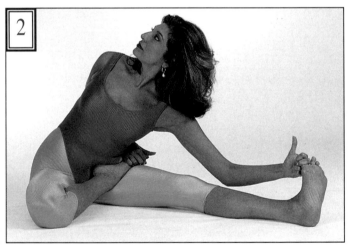

1

Place your left leg directly in front of your hip and your right foot on top of the left thigh, keeping hips and thighs down. Clasp your big toe.

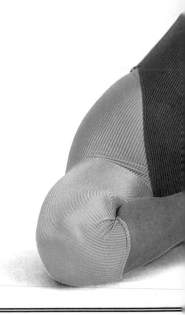

2

Twist the spine and look over your right shoulder. Take your right arm behind your back and clasp your right toes. Push thighs and knees down onto the floor and flex the big toe of your left leg back.

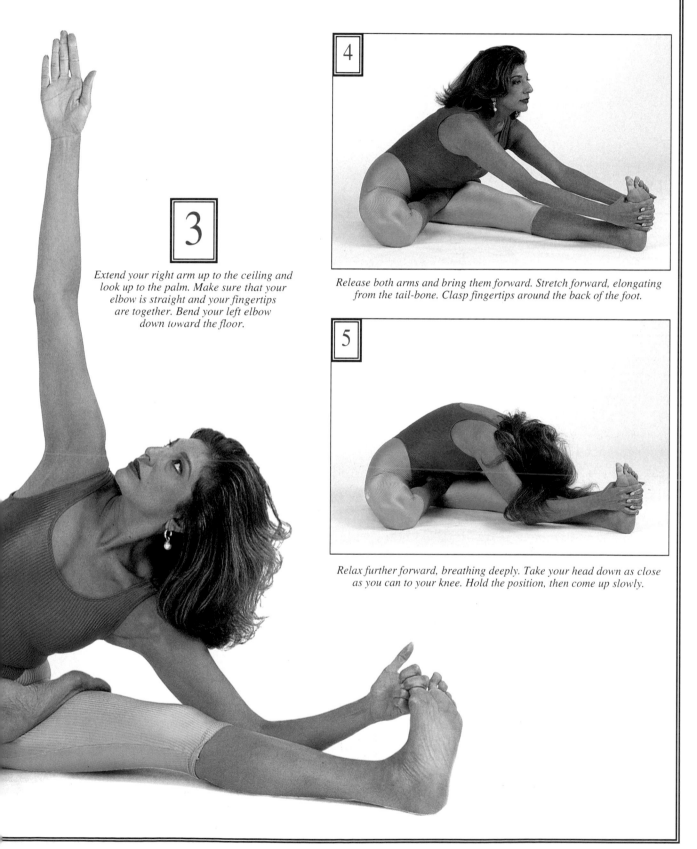

3

Extend your right arm up to the ceiling and look up to the palm. Make sure that your elbow is straight and your fingertips are together. Bend your left elbow down toward the floor.

4

Release both arms and bring them forward. Stretch forward, elongating from the tail-bone. Clasp fingertips around the back of the foot.

5

Relax further forward, breathing deeply. Take your head down as close as you can to your knee. Hold the position, then come up slowly.

Lying Flat Twist

This gentle twist relaxes the entire spinal column. It alleviates back pain and helps to prevent other back ailments such as sciatica and lumbago. Bring your knees up as close as possible to the arms to increase the spinal stretch. By keeping the shoulders flat on the floor and twisting the head in the opposite direction, an added stretch is felt in the neck, shoulders, upper and lower back and in the tail-bone. Always keep your knees together and tighten the abdominal muscles as you twist from side to side.

1

Starting with Step 1 of Deep Relaxation (see page 124), inhale and bring your knees toward the chest, keeping your lower legs parallel with the floor. Stretch your arms to the sides with palms face-down. Look up and relax the neck and shoulders. Keep your mouth closed and relax the jaw muscles.

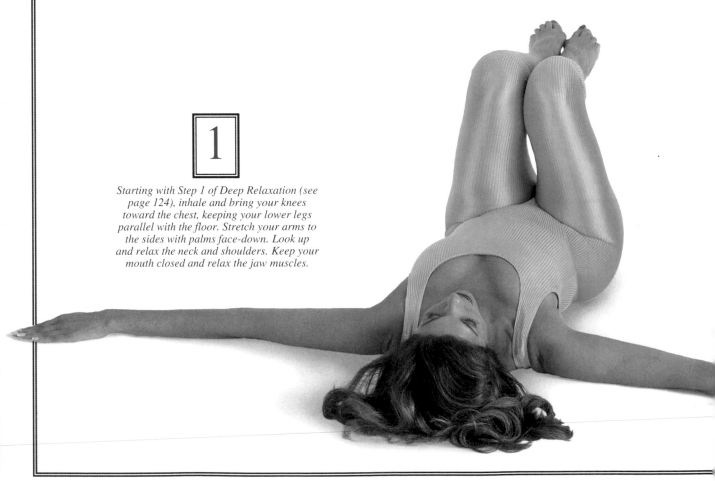

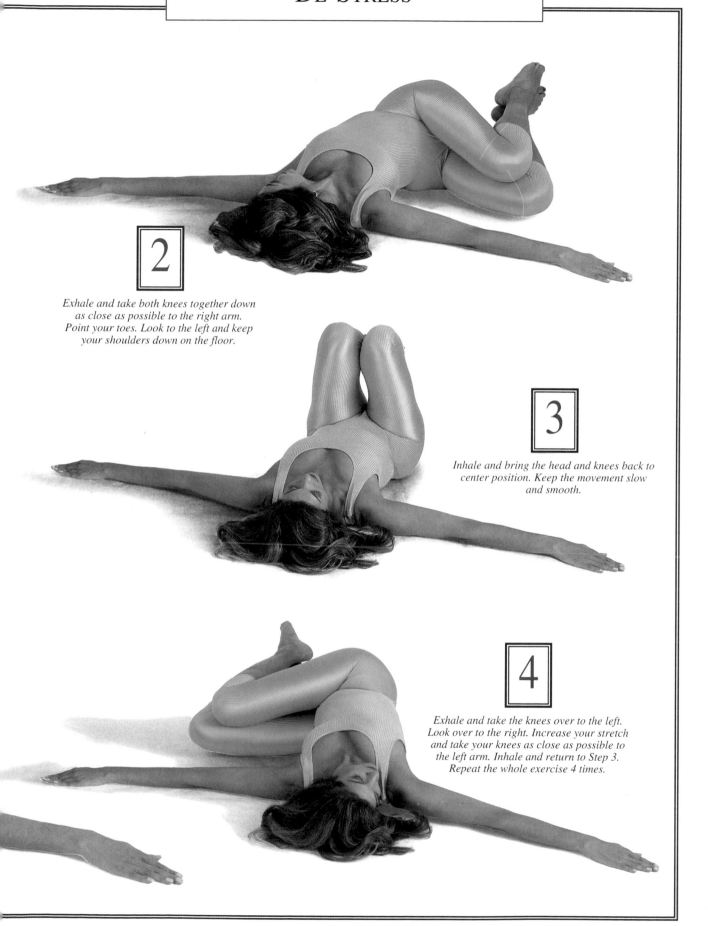

2

Exhale and take both knees together down as close as possible to the right arm. Point your toes. Look to the left and keep your shoulders down on the floor.

3

Inhale and bring the head and knees back to center position. Keep the movement slow and smooth.

4

Exhale and take the knees over to the left. Look over to the right. Increase your stretch and take your knees as close as possible to the left arm. Inhale and return to Step 3. Repeat the whole exercise 4 times.

The Camel

This intense back stretch invigorates the entire spine and expands the rib cage, allowing the lungs to breathe more deeply. The Camel also improves flexibility in the neck and spine and strengthens the lower back muscles, helping to relieve backache. Remember to push the hips forward as much as possible, increasing your stamina and strength. Opening the chest wide will create a positive attitude and to help you attain dynamic control over your whole body. Hold the final position for 10 seconds and raise yourself slowly.

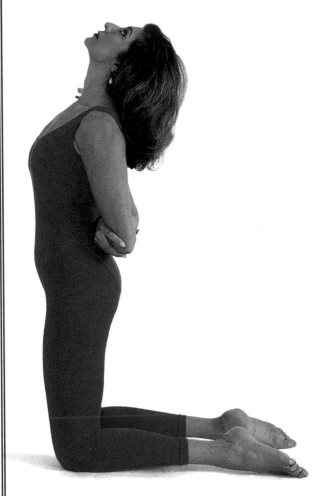

1

Kneel with your legs vertically under the hip bones. Look up and cross your arms over your lower back. Hold for 30 seconds.

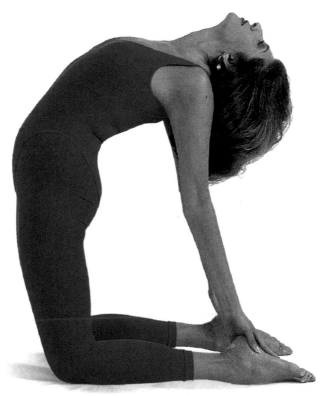

2

Inhale deeply and push your hips forward as you drop your arms down. Relax your neck and throat. Hold for 30 seconds.

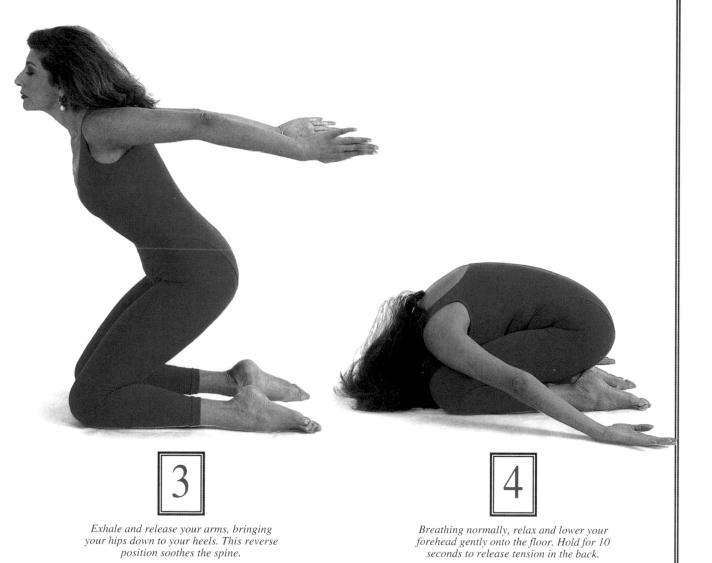

3

*Exhale and release your arms, bringing
your hips down to your heels. This reverse
position soothes the spine.*

4

*Breathing normally, relax and lower your
forehead gently onto the floor. Hold for 10
seconds to release tension in the back.*

The Rabbit

The Rabbit pose is used in *Hatha* Yoga as a preliminary exercise to the Head Stand. It stretches the spine, improving elasticity and mobility, and allows the nervous system to receive a good supply of fresh oxygen. The Rabbit also aids digestion and helps to prevent common colds, sinus problems and chronic tonsillitis. It has a wonderfully beneficial effect on the thyroid, which regulates the metabolism and helps to protect the body against toxins.

The placement of the head which carries about 25 per cent of your weight in Step 5 (the rest of your weight should be evenly distributed across your body) stimulates the pituitary gland, helping to ward off senility and keep you feeling youthful. Having held this final position for 20 seconds, you should uncurl slowly and return in exact reverse order to Step 1, then repeat the whole exercise one more time.

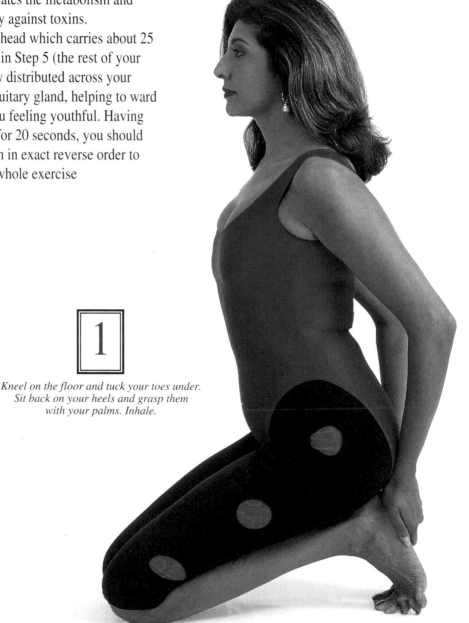

1

Kneel on the floor and tuck your toes under.
Sit back on your heels and grasp them
with your palms. Inhale.

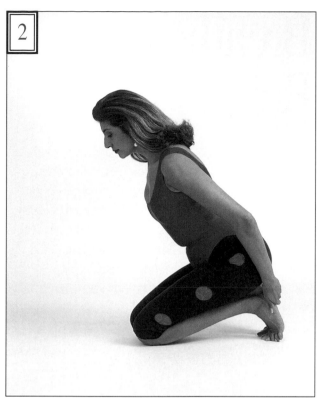

Exhale and slowly release forward at a 45° angle. Keep the
spine straight and tuck the stomach muscles in.

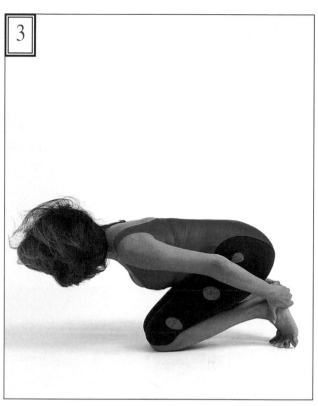

Inhale and hold when back is exactly flat and parallel to the floor.
Keep the toes firmly down, pushing the little toe into the floor.

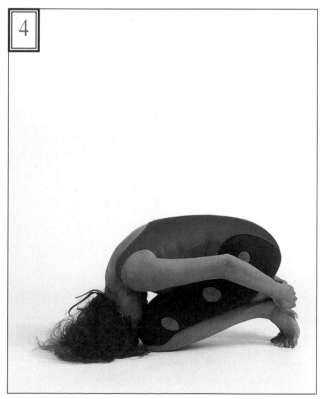

Exhale and curl your torso slowly forward to bring your forehead
as close as you can to your knees. Start breathing normally.

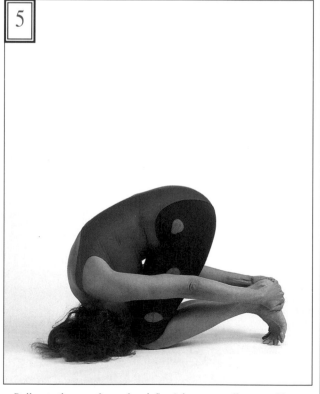

Roll onto the top of your head. Straighten your elbows and keep
curling forward with your hips upward. Hold for 20 seconds.

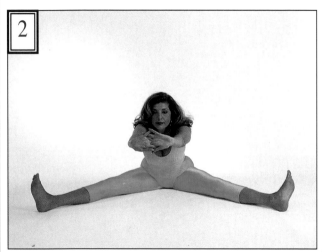

Sit up tall in wide 2nd position with knees flat on the floor. Flex the toes up. Inhale and stretch the arms over your head. Keep elbows straight, clasp fingertips together and look at the ceiling.

Breathe and Relax

Deep breathing is like a natural tranquilizer. It soothes the nervous system and helps you to increase your stretch by bringing the body weight into play. Do not bounce or force muscles as this will cause unnecessary strain. Just breathe and relax and discover the challenge of getting your chest and forehead right down to the floor. Hold every position for 5 seconds.

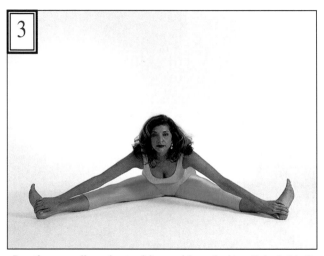

Exhale and stretch your arms straight out at shoulder level in front of you. Do not roll the hips forward and keep your buttock muscles down.

Breathe normally and extend forward from the hips. Take hold of your heels. If you cannot reach them, hold the thighs, knees or ankles. Keep your knees straight and your back flat.

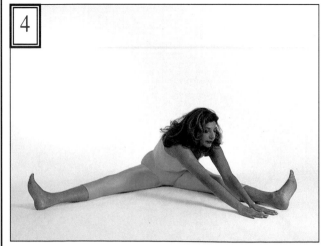

To increase the stretch, place both hands near the left foot. Stretch out as far as you can without rolling your hips and feet. Inhale and exhale slowly and continue to breathe normally.

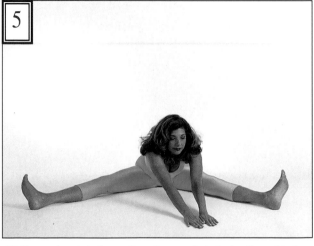

Walk your hands in front of you in a semi-circle, leading with the right hand. The inner side of your thighs will begin to loosen as the lower back and buttocks extend forward.

6

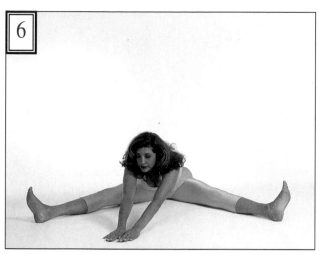

Keep lengthening through the center of your body. This boosts circulation to the pelvic region, stimulates the ovaries and helps to regulate the menstrual cycle.

7

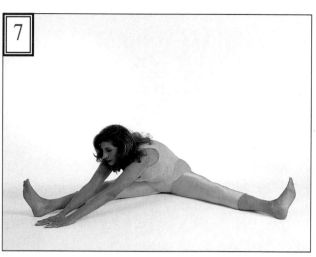

Move your hands across to your right leg. Do not let your hips rise off the floor and keep pushing your kneecaps down so that no light is visible between your legs and the floor.

8

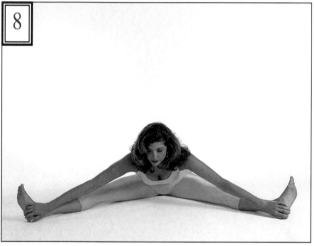

Take hold of both feet and each time you exhale, extend from the tail-bone and hips. Keep your shoulders relaxed. Continue to inhale and exhale slowly.

9

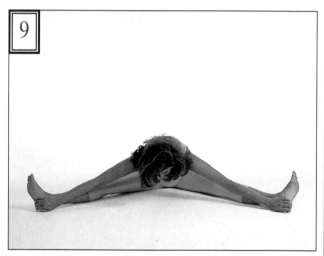

As you release forward on the exhalation, imagine all the tension leaving your body. As you relax you will find yourself stretching even more. Do not worry if you cannot reach the floor.

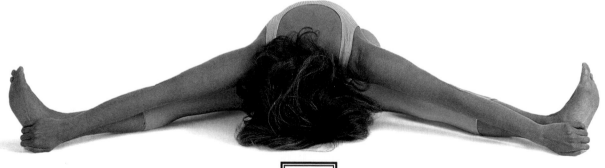

10

Keep the breathing even. Try to touch the floor with your chest and forehead. Hold for 10 seconds, then slowly release to a sitting position. Bring your legs together slowly and give them a shake.

Nerve Soother

This breathing technique massages and cleanses the abdominal organs. It helps to regulate bowel movements and strengthens the abdominal wall. Mental concentration improves as you coordinate the exhalation of a vigorous breath from your lips and a contraction of your abdominal muscles. Do not move any other part of your body, especially your arms, shoulders or lower back. Focus only on your stomach and think of all that fresh oxygen revitalizing the body. Start the exercise by sitting tall (as in Step 2), with arms straight, elbows turned out and hands on your knees for support.

1

Inhale deeply and slowly through your nose. Exhale through your mouth and blow vigorously through your lips as if blowing out a candle. Simultaneously contract and pull the stomach muscles in as you exhale. Curve the spine.

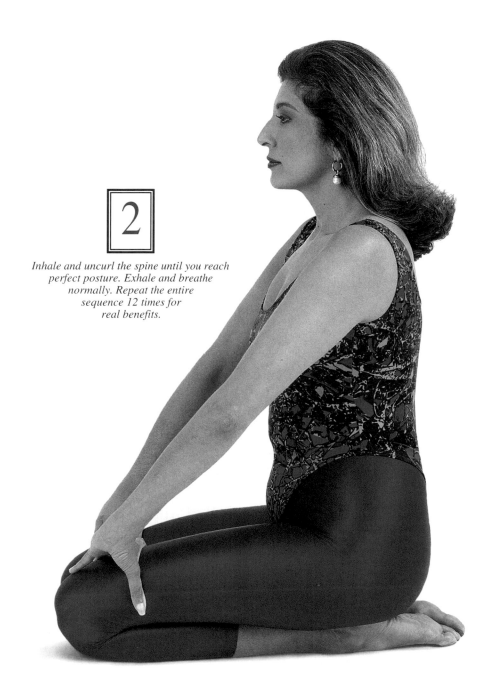

2

Inhale and uncurl the spine until you reach perfect posture. Exhale and breathe normally. Repeat the entire sequence 12 times for real benefits.

Deep Relaxation

This deep relaxation technique, often referred to as the 'Dead Man's Pose', replenishes valuable *prana,* or energy, that is lost through physical, emotional or mental exertion. Any uncontrolled emotions such as anger, anxiety, sorrow or greed quickly deplete our store of energy reserves. Mental exhaustion also causes strain in the muscles and imbalance in the internal organs. However, complete tranquility calms and soothes the

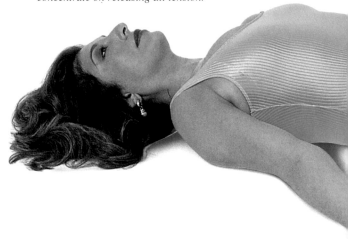

Lie on the floor or on a bed with palms up and feet relaxed. Breathe deeply through the nose from the diaphragm. As you exhale, concentrate on releasing all tension.

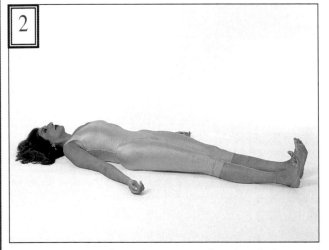

Concentrate on your feet and toes, moving them first clockwise and anti-clockwise, then pointing them down to the floor as hard as you can (as illustrated in Step 4).

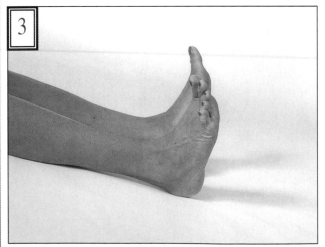

Flex your toes and heels upward and tighten the ankles, lower legs, knees, thighs, stomach and buttocks. Then releasing slowly from the toes, relax all joints and muscles below the waist.

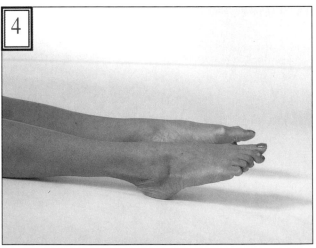

Rotate your feet clockwise and anti-clockwise again (as in Step 2), then point your toes down to the floor as hard as you can. Now repeat Step 3.

nerves, regulates blood pressure, boosts the body's circulation and rejuvenates every cell in the body. The relaxation technique demonstrated here and on the following pages works on three levels: the physical, mental and the spiritual. It teaches you how to isolate the problem muscle groups and by tensing and relaxing the muscles in turn, guides you through the deepest level of relaxation to reduce stress and fatigue.

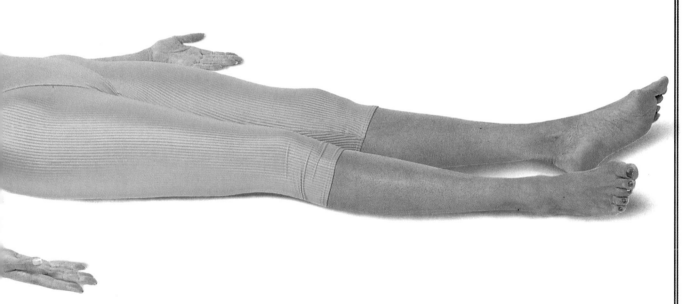

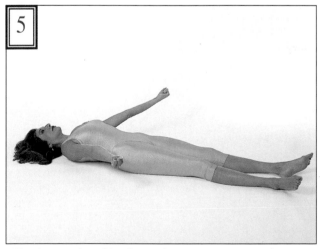

5

Keeping your breathing deep and even, concentrate on the upper body, especially the hands, arms and shoulders. Inhale, clench your fists and raise arms 30cm (1ft) off the floor.

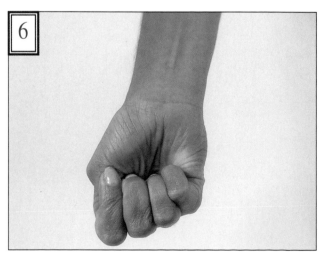

6

Clench your raised fists as tightly as possible to flex the hands, arms, elbows and shoulders. Keep the elbows straight. Hold for 5 seconds.

The mind thus becomes still, allowing you to escape from the problems of everyday life. Mentally withdrawing yourself from your body enables you to identify with your higher consciousness and can bring inner peace and joy.

This exercise can be done during the day to rejuvenate the mind and body or at night to relax you for sleep. If you perform this exercise in bed at night you will most probably fall asleep. If you do it during the day, try to keep yourself awake but in a dreamy trance. Slowly 'come back to life' after 15 minutes. Begin by moving your toes and fingertips, and feel the energy flow through your entire body. When you feel like getting up, take your arms over behind your head, stretch your fingers and toes, then slowly sit up tall.

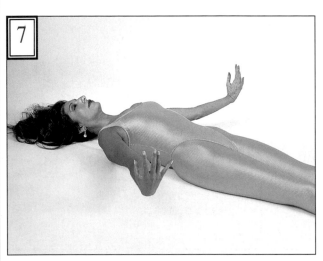

Exhale. Release and relax the hands, arms, elbows and shoulders and lower your hands with upturned palms onto the floor.

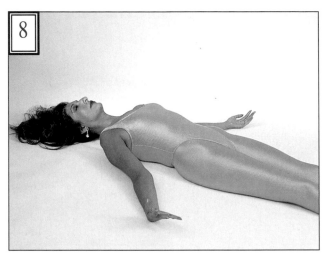

Now start to concentrate on releasing tension from your neck and shoulders. Breathe normally for 5 seconds.

11

Try to push all disturbing thoughts from your mind so that it becomes still and calm. As you exhale, imagine you are on a cloud and completely weightless.

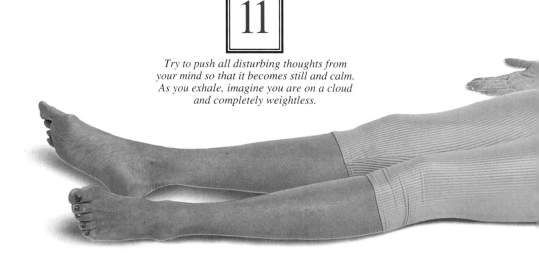

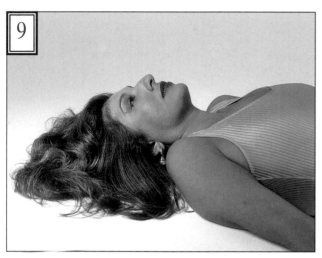

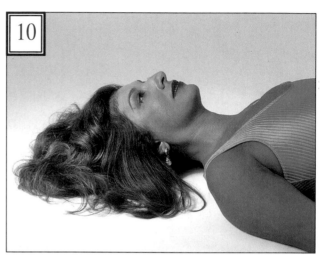

Bring both shoulders up toward your ears as shown, then exhale and relax them down. Repeat until you feel all tension disappear from this area.

Roll your head from side to side, letting it rest wherever comfortable. Now concentrate on the muscles in the face. Relax the jaw, and the muscles around the eyes and forehead.

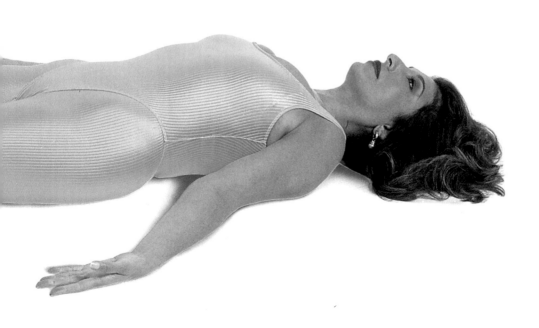

ACKNOWLEDGEMENTS

COMMISSIONING EDITOR: SIAN FACER

EDITORS: JANE MCINTOSH SUSIE BEHAR

ART EDITOR: KEITH MARTIN

ART DIRECTOR: JACQUI SMALL

DESIGNER: PAUL CARPENTER

PRODUCTION: ANTONIA MCARDLE

PHOTOGRAPHY: JOHN ADRIAAN

HAIRSTYLING: JOSEPH ROBERTS

MAKEUP: TRACY WELLS

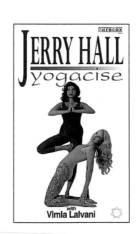